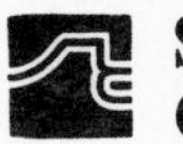

An Illustrated Guide to

Human Reproduction & Fertility Control

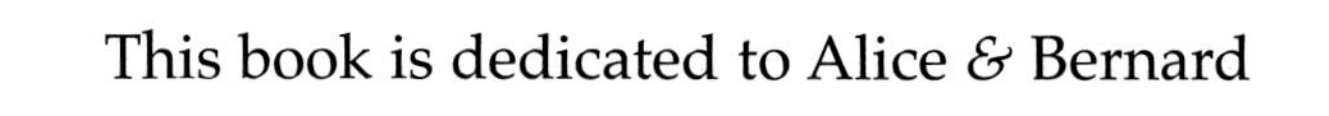

This book is dedicated to Alice & Bernard

AN ILLUSTRATED GUIDE TO

Human Reproduction & Fertility Control

Robert J. Demarest, CMI
Director, Center for Biomedical Communications (Retired)
College of Physicians & Surgeons
Columbia University, New York, NY, USA

&

Rita Charon, MD
Associate Professor of Clinical Medicine
College of Physicians & Surgeons
Columbia University, New York, NY, USA

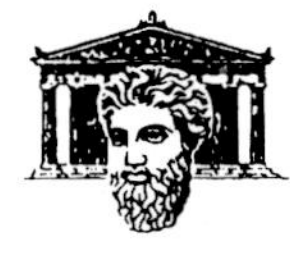

The Parthenon Publishing Group
INTERNATIONAL PUBLISHERS IN MEDICINE, SCIENCE & TECHNOLOGY
NEW YORK LONDON

Library of Congress Cataloging-in-Publication Data
Demarest, Robert J.
Illustrated Guide to Human Reproduction & Fertility Control / Robert J. Demarest and Rita Charon.
p. cm.
ISBN 1-85070-697-2
1. Pregnancy. 2. Childbirth. 3. Human Reproduction. I. Charon, Rita. II. Title.
RG525.D35 1995
612.6--dc60
95-23415
CIP

British Library Cataloguing in Publication Data
Demarest, Robert J.
Illustrated Guide to Human Reproduction & Fertility Control.
I. Title. II. Charon, Rita
618.2

ISBN 1-85070-697-2

Published in North America by
The Parthenon Publishing Group Inc.
One Blue Hill Plaza
Pearl River
New York 10965, USA

Published in the UK and Europe by
The Parthenon Publishing Group Limited
Casterton Hall, Carnforth
Lancs. LA6 2LA, UK

First published 1996

Cover design by Matthew Doherty Design, Evanston, IL, USA
Interior design by Kenneth Turbeville, Waco, TX, USA
Printed and bound by T.G. Hostench S.A., Spain

Table of Contents

Authors' Note

Issues of conception, birth, and birth control engage all women and men. The decision to have a baby is probably the most momentous decision a woman or a man can make. In addition, effective birth control, overpopulation, abortion, and infertility are important subjects for personal and public discussion. All of us must join in this conversation, not only the scientists with specialized knowledge about reproduction or spokespeople on one side or the other of the political debates, but all members of the global community. This book offers accessible information about the anatomy of men and women, the physiological steps that lead to conception and gestation and birth, and the means we have to control these events. Our understanding of these marvelous processes, however, is always incomplete, so any book of medical information will contain uncertainties and tentative truths. We hope that high school and college students, young adults, men and women facing decisions about fertility, and the clinicians who care for them will use this book's illustrations and text to pierce the mystery and misinformation that sometimes surround these issues, realizing that a book cannot replace the education and counsel of the individual doctor or nurse. With clear knowledge in hand, all of us can make informed decisions and take appropriate actions regarding our own fertility and humane reproductive policies throughout the world.

We thank Dr. Tessie Tharakan, Assistant Professor of Obstetrics and Gynecology of Columbia University, for her expert and thoughtful consultation throughout the writing of this book. Thanks also to Ilan E. Timor, M.D.,Director of Obstetrical Service & Ob/Gyn Ultrasound and Professor of Clinical Obstetrics and Gynecology, Columbia University for supplying the ultrasound pictures.

Robert J. Demarest

Rita Charon, M.D.

Introduction

The birth of a new baby is the culmination of many complex events. First, the egg develops in the mother's ovary and the sperm develops in the father's testicle. Both the egg and the sperm contain the parent's chromosomes, endowing a future child with the characteristics of the parent, the grandparents, and even the great-grandparents. Then, in the act of sexual intercourse, the father's sperm travels through his penis into the mother's vagina to be brought close to the waiting egg. If the egg and sperm meet in the step called fertilization and if the mother's uterus is prepared for pregnancy, the joined cells may come to rest, or be implanted, within the lining of the uterus. There, with nourishment from the pregnant mother, the cells grow into the embryo and then the fetus. Finally, after nine months of wondrous growth and individuation, a child is born.

We are beginning to know a great deal about the development of egg and sperm, about the conditions that favor fertilization and implantation, and about the development of the fertilized egg into a new human being. Some of this knowledge allows couples to practice birth control, to have a child despite evidence of infertility, or to terminate a pregnancy already begun. There is still much to learn. Why are some pregnancies lost in miscarriages or stillbirths? Why do some couples have trouble conceiving a child? How are the rates of fertility influenced by such global factors as drought, crowding, economic shifts, or discord?

Even though scientists may learn about all the details of the reproductive cycles of women and men and the physiological events that lead to birth, all humans remain in awe of their miraculous abilities to take part in the creation of new life. By taking readers step-by-step through the development of egg and sperm, fertilization, implantation, embryonic and fetal growth, and birth as well as methods of birth control, termination of pregnancy, treatment for infertile couples, and menopause, this book hopes to contribute to both the knowledge and the awe that surround human reproduction.

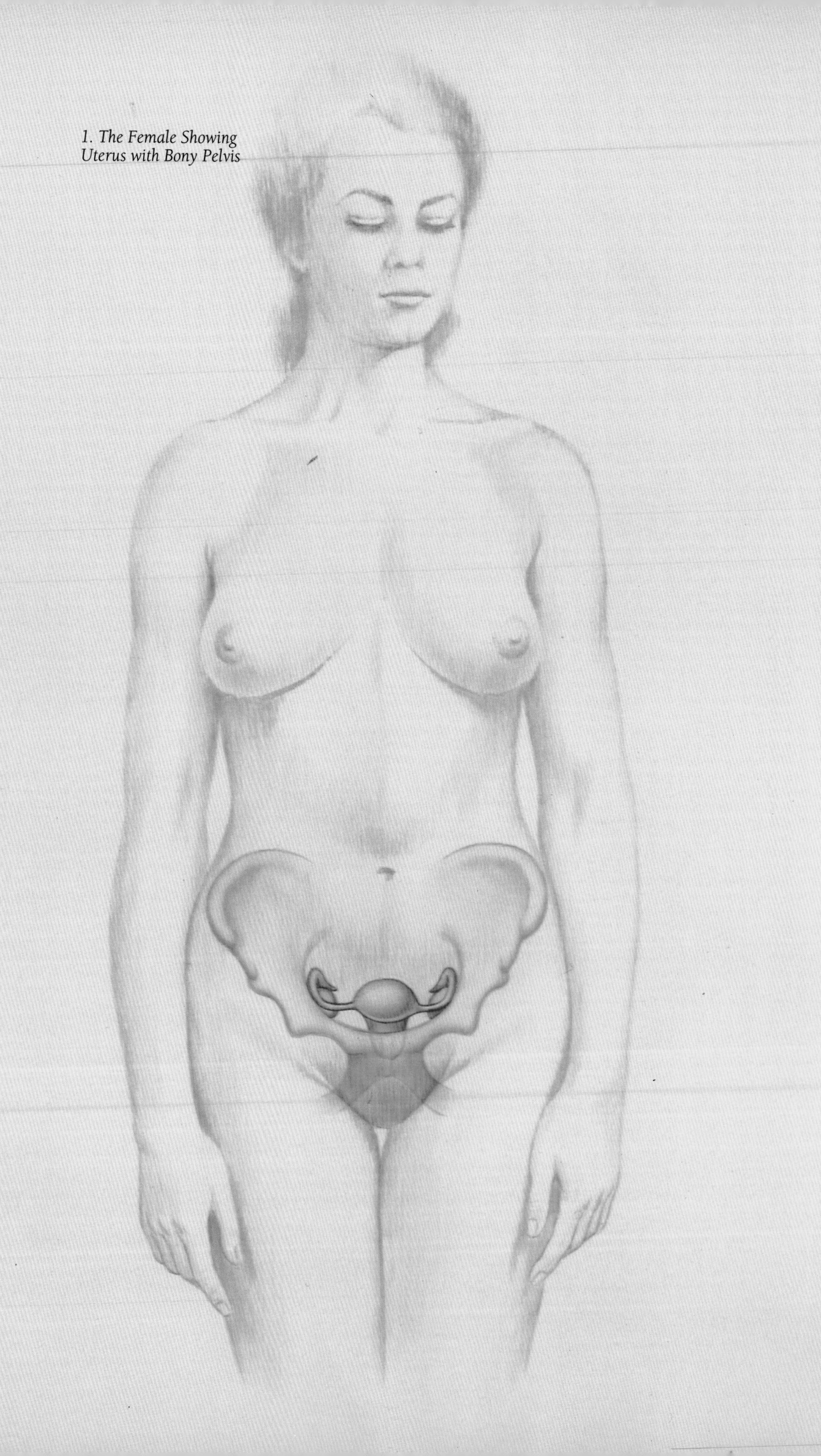

1. The Female Showing Uterus with Bony Pelvis

On the Woman's Side: Reproductive Anatomy

From the time a woman's menstrual cycle begins in adolescence until it ceases in menopause, her body prepares for pregnancy every month unless she is already pregnant, breast-feeding, or taking birth-control pills. Many organs of her body–the hypothalamus and the pituitary gland in her brain, the ovaries and uterus in her abdomen, her breasts, and her vagina have a role to play in reproduction.

The female reproductive system includes external organs and internal reproductive organs. Together, they allow a woman to conceive and bear a child. The external organs allow intercourse and sexual pleasure, and the internal organs produce the egg and nurture the developing child.

External Reproductive Organs

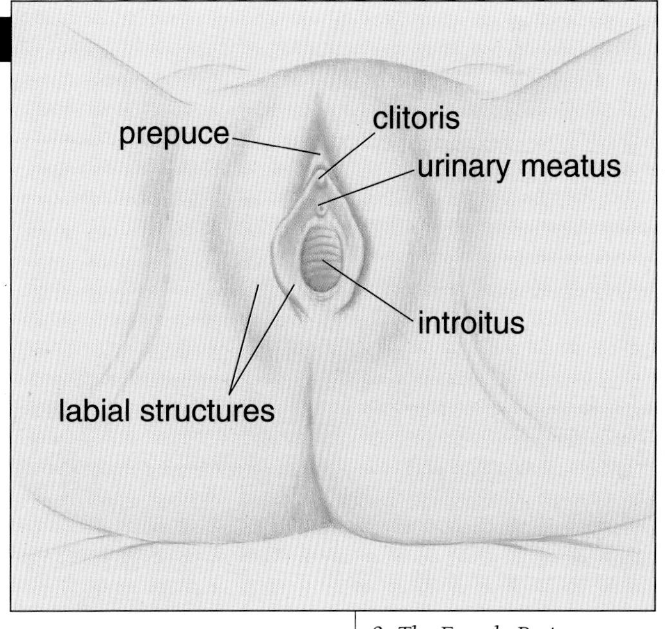

2. The Female Perineum

Collectively called the vulva, the external organs include the mons pubis, the labia majora, the labia minora, the clitoris, and the entrance to the vagina. The mons pubis is the soft cushion of tissue on top of the pelvic bones, called the pubic symphysis, at the front of the pelvic area. The mons pubis is covered with pubic hair once a female reaches puberty. The opening to the vagina, or introitus, is surrounded by two pairs of lips. The labia majora are the outer, larger lips. They, too, are covered with hair in mature women. Under the labia majora are two smaller lips called the labia minora. Within the folds of the labia under a protective covering called the prepuce is the clitoris. Formed of erectile tissue similar to the penis in the male, the pearl-shaped clitoris is richly supplied with nerves that give erotic pleasure to the woman. The clitoris is important in sexuality and reproduction, for its stimulation leads to the sublime pleasures of arousal and orgasm.

Below the clitoris is the urinary meatus, the opening for urine to pass from the bladder to the outside. Around the clitoris and the urinary meatus are pairs of glands–the Bartholin glands and the Skene glands–that release lubricating fluids during arousal and intercourse.

The vagina is a muscular canal that leads from the vulva to the uterus. During intercourse, the man's penis enters the vagina. As a woman becomes aroused and reaches orgasm, her vagina contracts rhythmically, both giving her pleasure and propelling the man's emission toward her cervix.

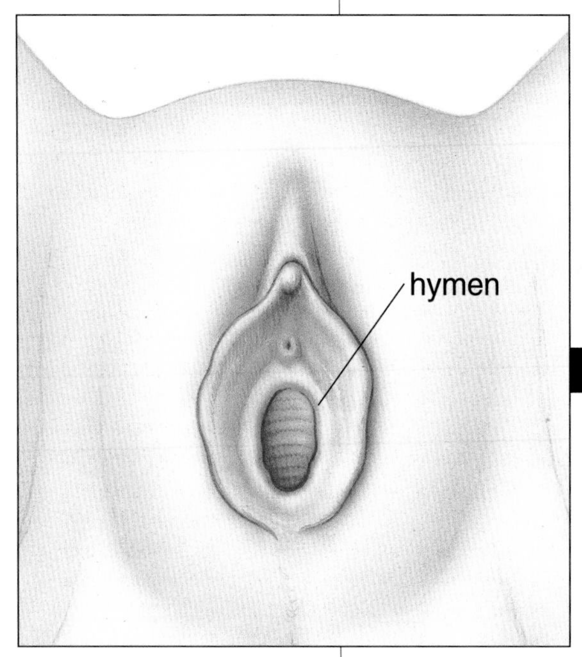

3. *Intact Hymen as it Appears in the Young Female*

Girls' vaginal openings are covered with the hymen, a membrane of variable thickness through which menstrual flow can pass. Although the hymen is disturbed when intercourse takes place, the hymen of a virgin can look similar to that of a woman who has had intercourse, making the so-called rupture of the hymen more myth than reality.

INTERNAL REPRODUCTIVE ORGANS

The internal reproductive organs include the ovaries, the Fallopian tubes or oviducts, the uterus, and the cervix. These organs are held within the bones of the pelvis. Because a baby must have room to grow and to be born, a woman's pelvic bones are different from a man's—fuller in the hips and wider at the bottom. The obstetrician will measure a pregnant woman's pelvic bones to assure that the baby will have room to pass through the outlet. Rarely, the bones are too narrow and a delivery has to be done through Cesarean section, or an incision in the uterine wall.

The ovaries are smooth, glistening, almond-shaped organs about one inch wide by one-and-a-half inches long that lie on either side of the uterus. They are sensitive to touch, and a woman will generally feel a twinge during a pelvic examination when her ovaries are examined by the doctor or nurse.

> ***"One egg every month develops a follicle, that is, a nest of tissue that nurtures the growing egg."***

Complex and ever changing, the ovaries contain hundreds of thousands of eggs, produce estrogen and other hormones, and usually release one egg every month for potential fertilization. No one knows why a girl child is born with around six hundred thousand eggs even though, over the course of her life, only around 500 will develop and be released. One egg every month develops a follicle, that is, a nest of tissue that nurtures the growing egg. Special growth factors produced by the ovary seem to select and support the egg and its follicle. The ovary's tissues also produce estrogen, progesterone, and androgen, the hormones that direct the events of pregnancy and delivery in the womb, the breasts, and the placenta.

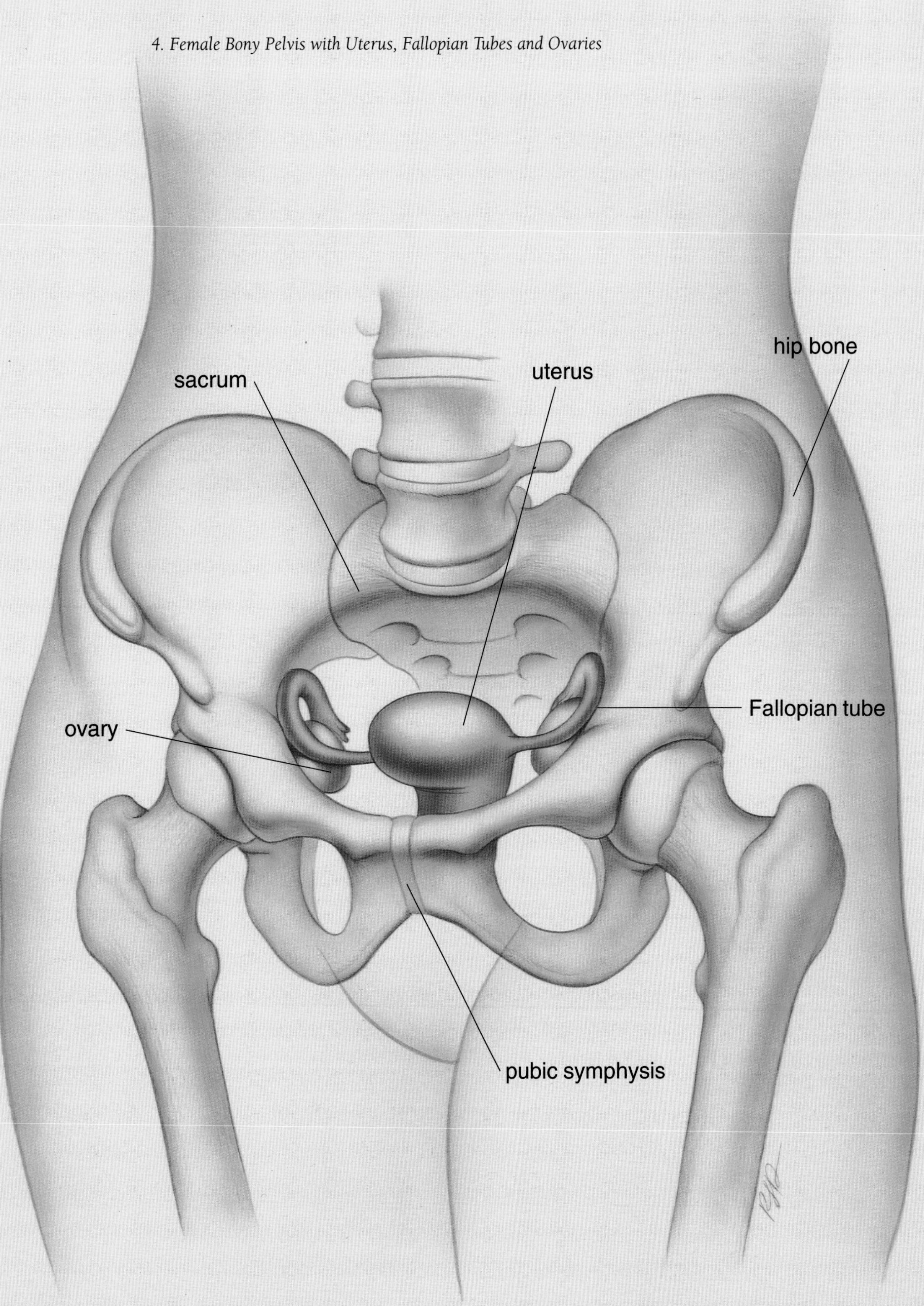

4. Female Bony Pelvis with Uterus, Fallopian Tubes and Ovaries

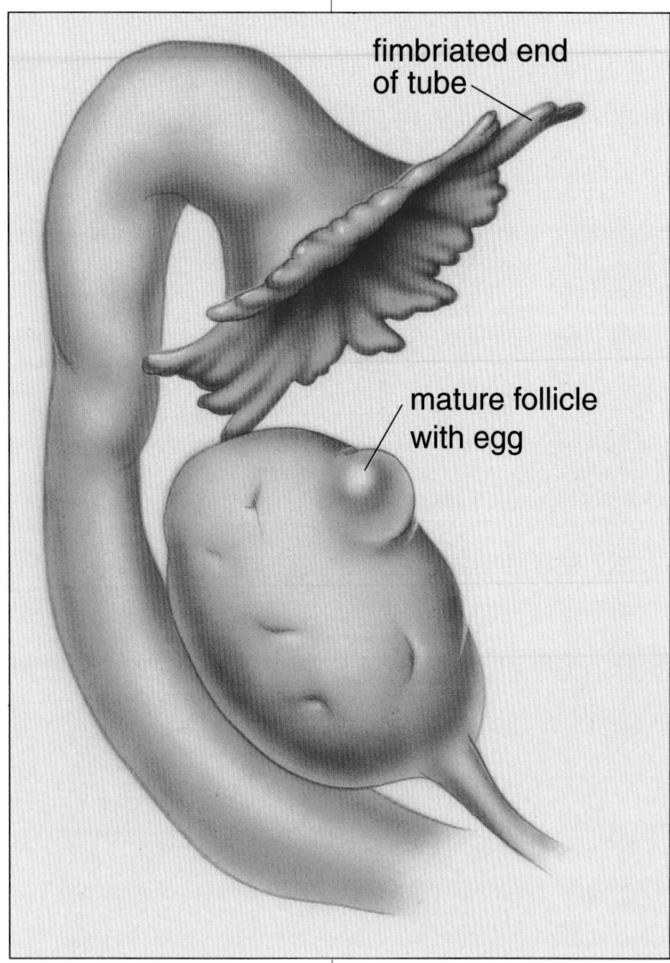

5. *Fallopian Tube and Ovary (enlarged)*

The ovary is loosely held by muscle tissue near the opening of the Fallopian tube. Also called the oviduct, this funnel-shaped tube reaches toward the ovary with its fringed opening and connects to the inside of the womb.

Around four to seven inches long, the Fallopian tube catches the egg when it is released from the surface of the ovary and directs it into the interior of the uterus. Illustration 6 shows an egg traveling down the Fallopian tube toward the womb. The muscles in the walls of the tube beat constantly, tightening and relaxing rhythmically to permit movement of the egg toward the womb. This tube is tied to prevent pregnancy in the tubal ligation procedure.

The uterus, or womb, is a pear-shaped organ in the center of the woman's pelvis, between the urinary bladder and the rectum. In a woman who has not been pregnant, the uterus is around three to four inches long, and after a woman has had children, the uterus can be around five inches long. When the woman is pregnant, though, the uterus grows to accommodate the infant, attaining a length of over a foot-and-a-half. The walls of the uterus are made of strong muscles so that the baby can be pushed out of the womb during labor and delivery. The cramps that many women experience with their periods are caused by the activity of the muscles in the uterus. The inside surface of the womb, called the endometrium, is spongy, bloody tissue that once a month prepares for the arrival of a fertilized egg. If a pregnancy does not develop, the lining of the uterus flows out in the menstrual period. The cervix is the narrow canal that connects the uterus to the vagina. When a woman has a pelvic examination, the speculum is placed in the vagina so the tip of the cervix can be examined.

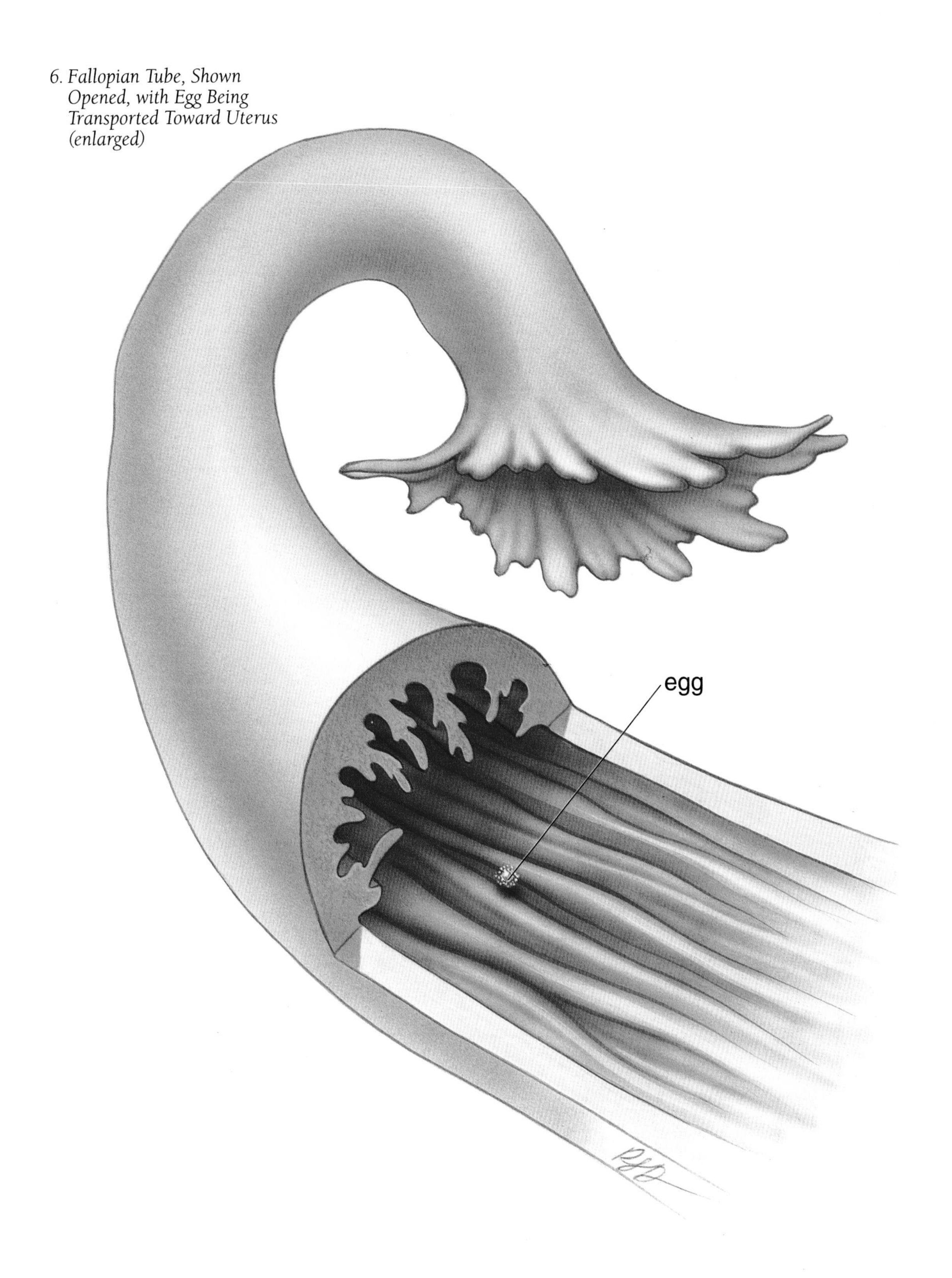

6. Fallopian Tube, Shown Opened, with Egg Being Transported Toward Uterus (enlarged)

7. Internal Female Reproductive Organs (actual size)

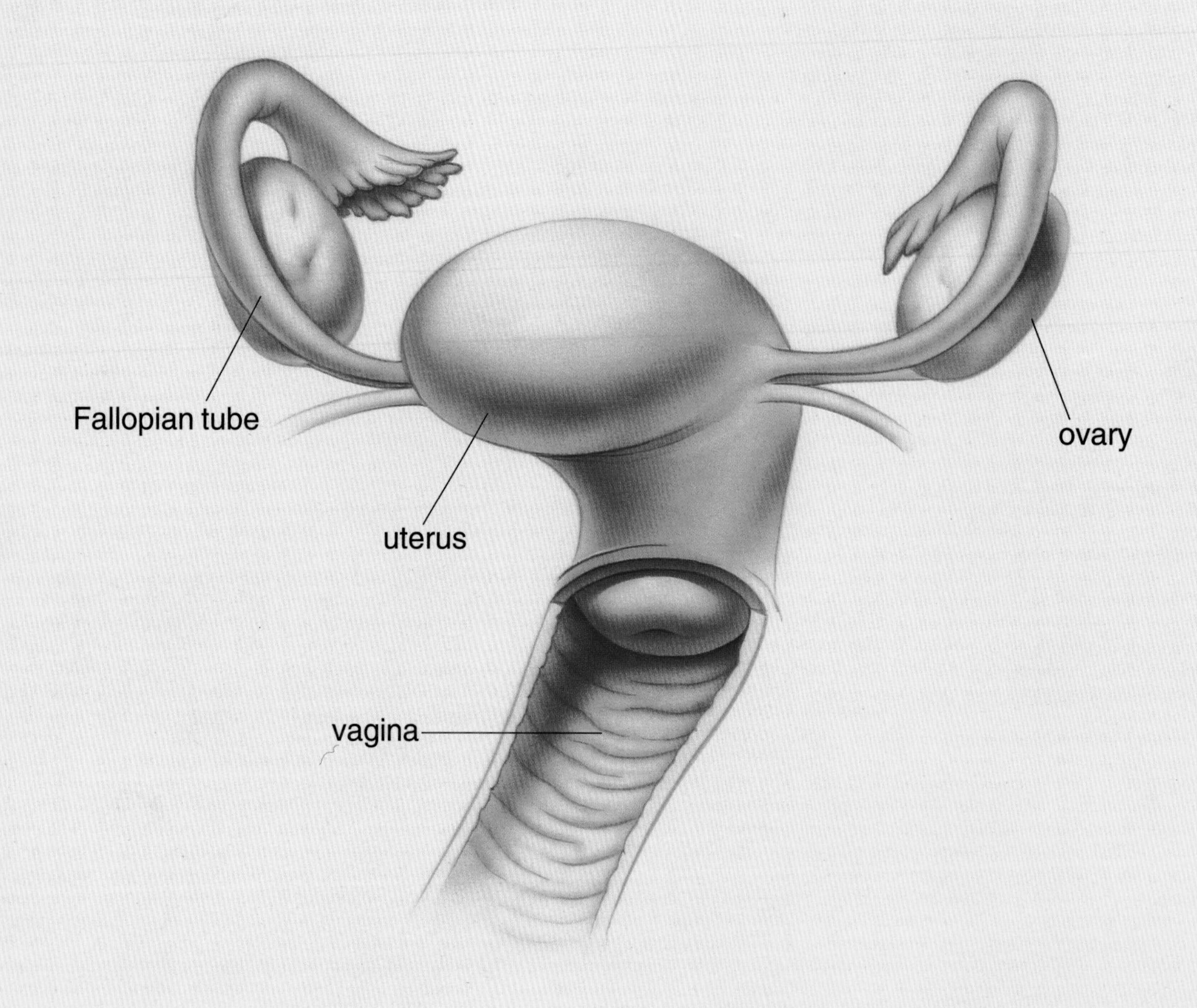

8. Cross Section of Uterus, Fallopian Tube and Ovary (actual size)

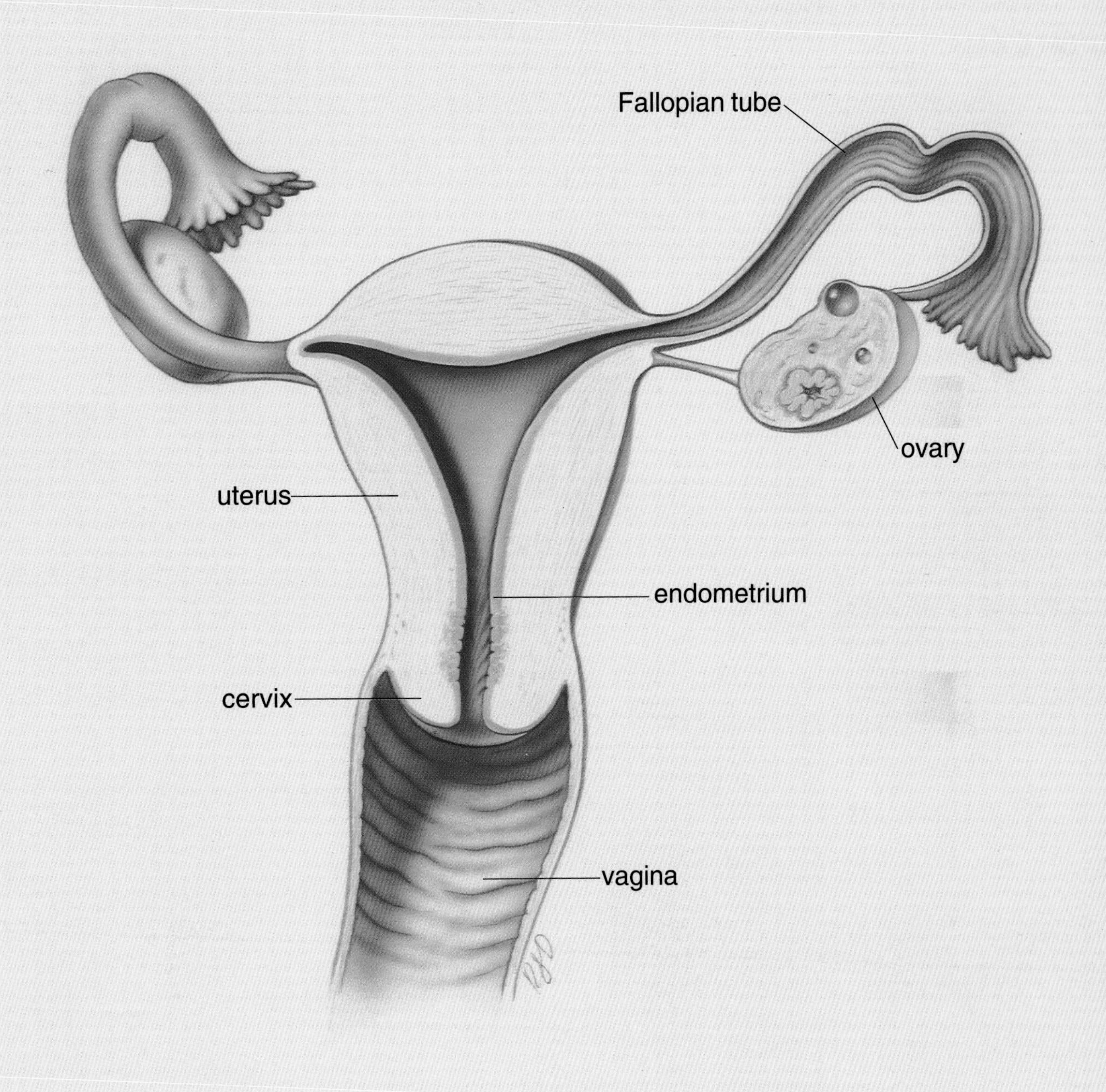

OTHER ORGANS OF REPRODUCTION

"The pituitary gland produces hormones called gonadotropins that direct the activities of the ovaries and follicles."

Several other organs in a woman's body take part in reproduction. The pituitary gland, a pea-sized gland in the center of the brain, produces hormones called gonadotropins that direct the activities of the ovaries and follicles. The breasts respond to the sex hormones and, if a woman is pregnant, begin to produce milk for feeding the infant. The nipples of the breast are surrounded with the areola, halos of sensitive skin that give the woman pleasure during sexual play. In both pregnancy and in sexual function, a woman's entire body–her muscles, her circulation, her breathing, her skin–contributes to her ability to reproduce and her capacity for pleasure.

9. Female Pelvic Organs Shown from the Side (partially sectioned)

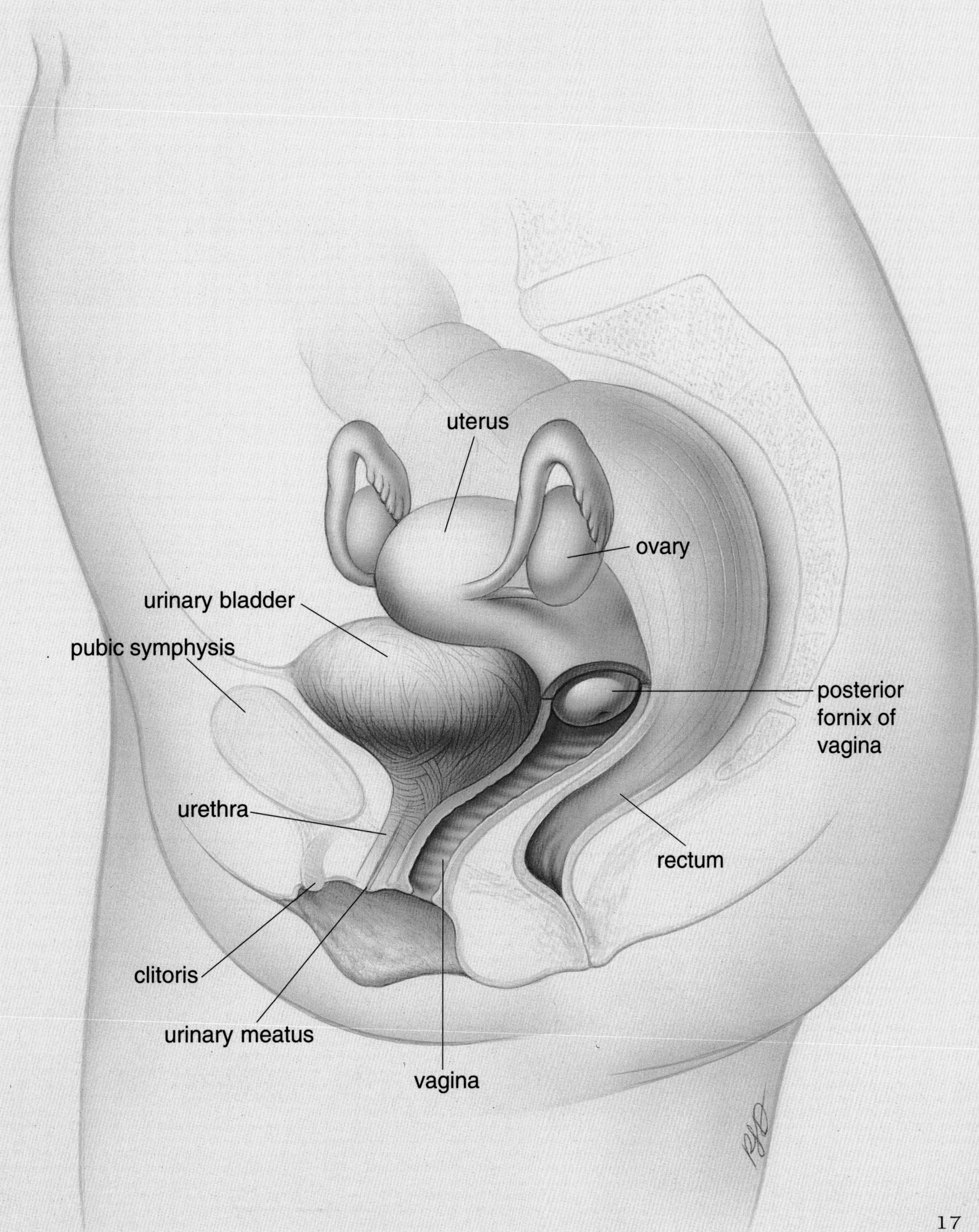

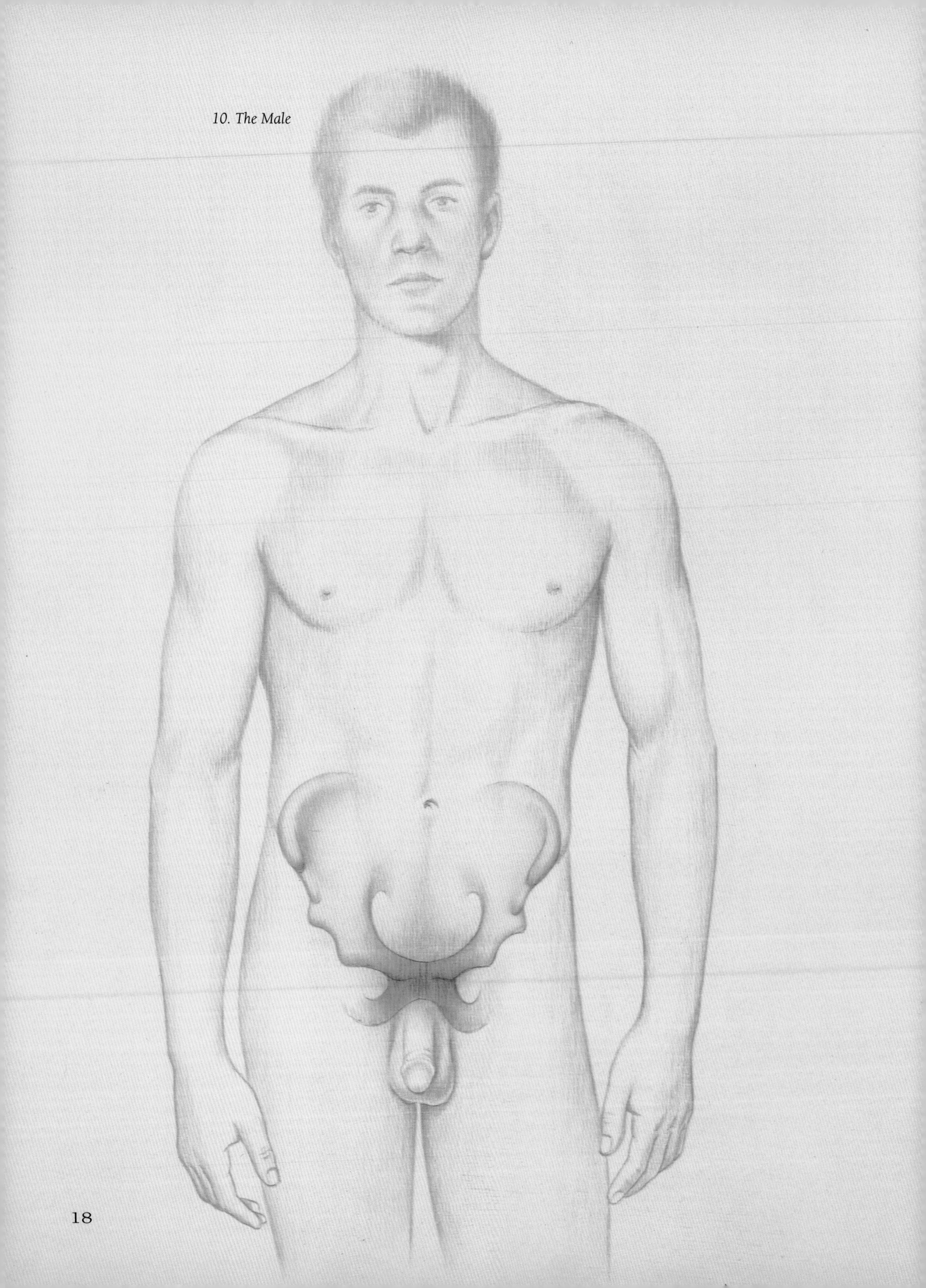

10. The Male

On the Man's Side: Reproductive Anatomy

The male's reproductive system is designed to deliver active healthy sperm cells into the woman's vagina so that, when an egg passes down her oviduct toward the uterus, the sperm can unite with it to begin a pregnancy. Unlike a woman, the man is always producing reproductive cells. He has no monthly cycle and his sperm is ready at every act of intercourse to lead to a pregnancy. Compared to a woman who releases around 500 eggs in her lifetime, the man releases approximately four or five million sperm cells each time he ejaculates, that is, ejects semen from the tip of the penis.

11. Male Reproductive Anatomy

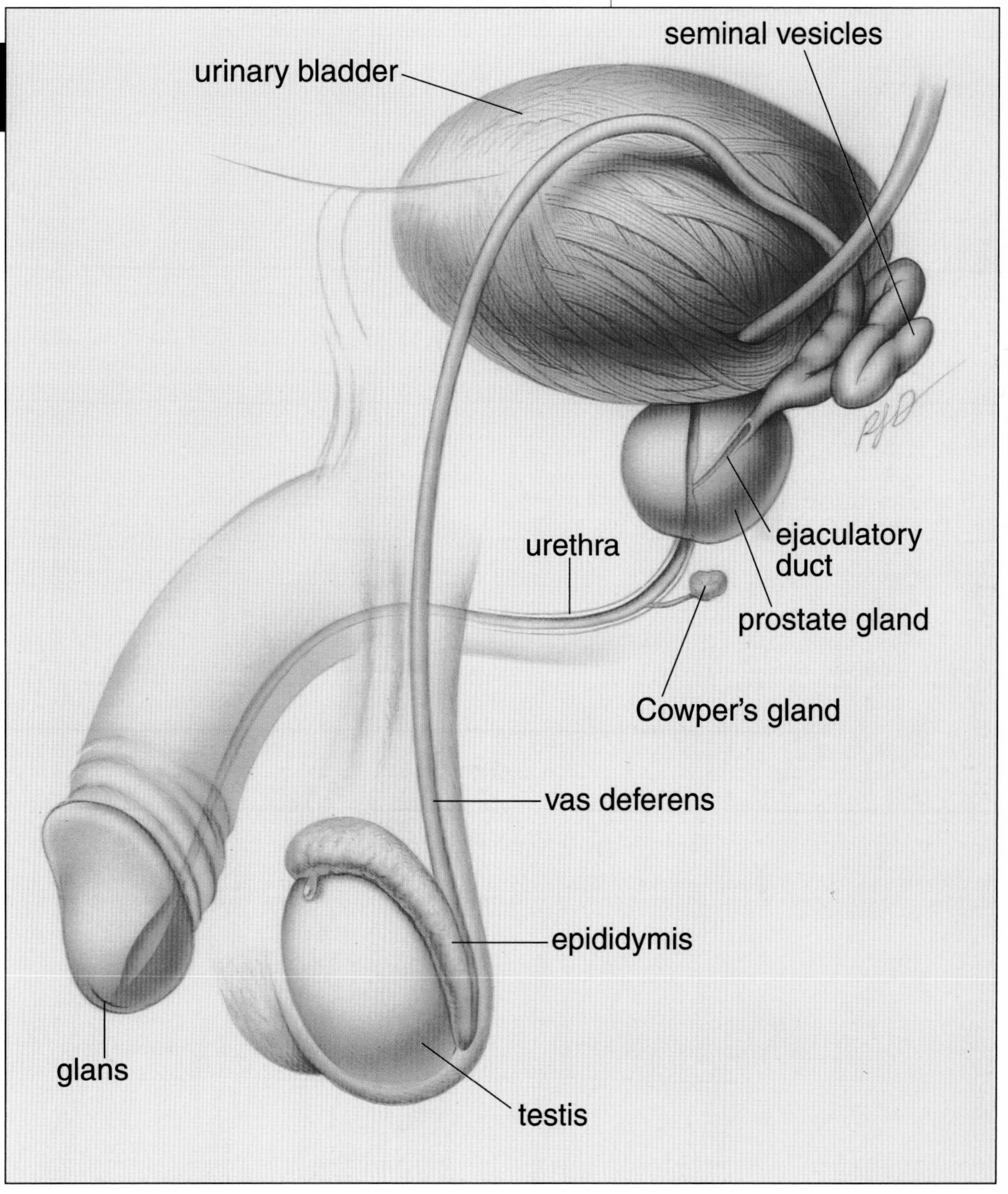

Reproductive Organs

The reproductive organs in the male are the testicles, the scrotal sac, the penis, and the ducts that carry the sperm and accompanying fluids through the penis and out of the body. The testicles, also called the testes, are the male's gonads. Paired, egg-shaped, and sensitive to touch, the testes lie outside the abdomen in the scrotal sac. Usually the left testis lies a little lower in the scrotal sac than does the right. Each testis is around one-and-a-half inches long and about one inch wide.

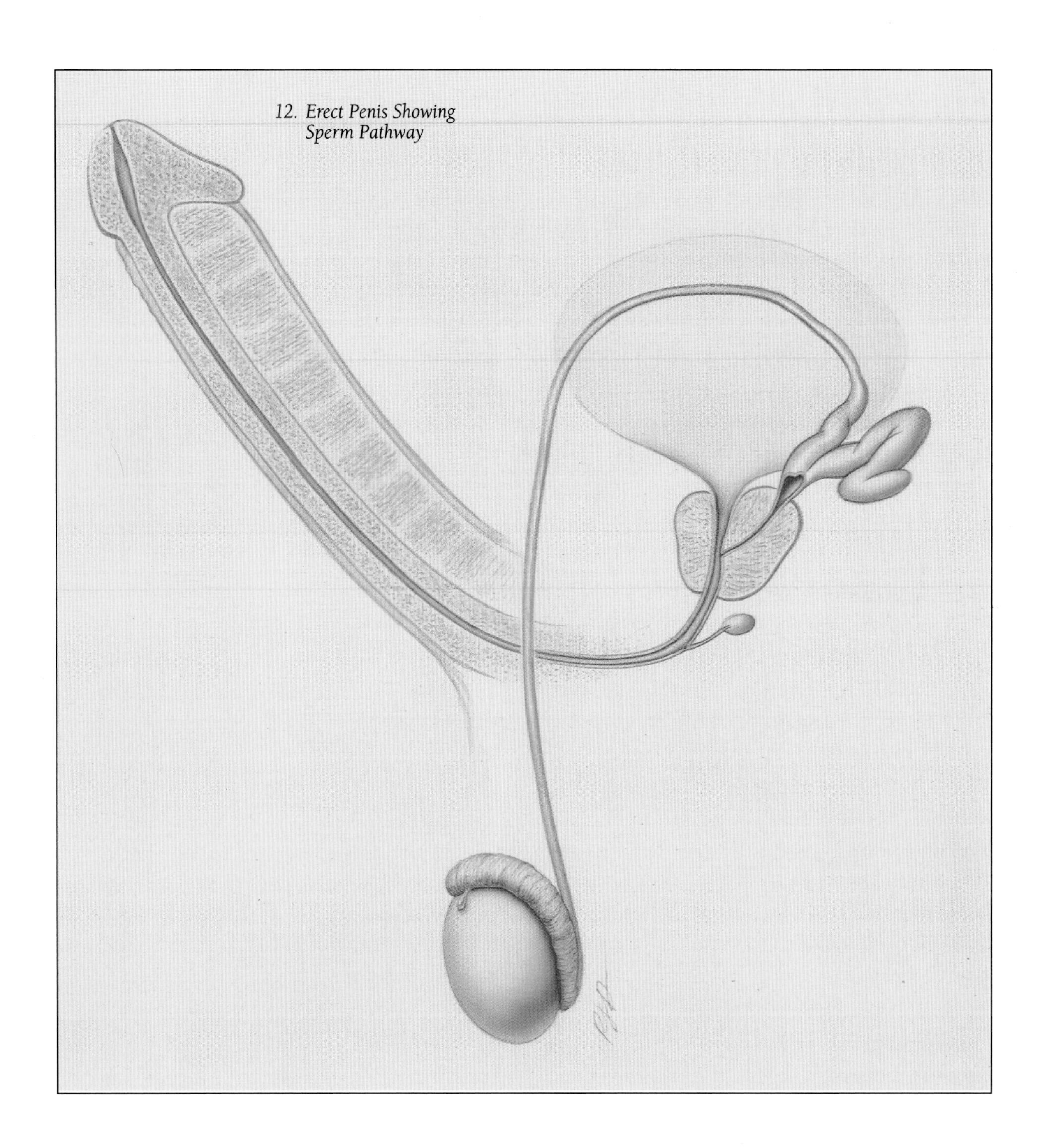
12. *Erect Penis Showing Sperm Pathway*

Within the tissue of the testes, sperm cells develop and the male hormones testosterone and dihydrotestosterone are produced.

A long, convoluted tube called the epididymis collects the sperm and testicular fluids and brings them toward the tip of the penis. Connected to the testis at the top surface and coiled very tightly, the epididymis not only stores sperm while waiting for ejaculation but also secretes fluids into the semen. If the epididymis were to be uncoiled, it would be around twenty feet long.

The end of the epididymis straightens out to form a tube called the vas deferens which, along with the spermatic cord carrying blood vessels and nerves, enters the lower abdomen. The vas deferens then hooks around the ureter as it enters the urinary bladder and empties into the urethra, the tube that carries urine from the bladder to the tip of the penis. Urine and semen take turns traveling in the urethra. At the point where the vas deferens enters the urethra, glands called the seminal vesicles add additional fluid to the semen. These glands also store semen between ejaculations. The prostate gland surrounds the urethra at the base of the penis, and it also contributes fluid to the semen before ejaculation.

The penis is composed of a root, a body or shaft, and a tip called the glans penis. When relaxed, the penis hangs in front of the testicles. When the man is aroused sexually, the erectile tissue of the penis becomes stiffly engorged with blood, nearly doubling in size. The prepuce, or foreskin, covers the glans penis unless it is removed by circumcision. In addition to being a conduit of urine and semen, the penis is a muscular organ, contracting with force on ejaculation of semen.

"Within the tissue of the testes, sperm cells develop and the male hormones testosterone and dihydrotestosterone are produced."

BRAIN, MIND, AND BODY

As in the female, other parts of a man's body play a role in reproduction. The hypothalamus and pituitary gland in the brain release hormones that activate sperm production and testosterone release. A man's emotional state and stress level influence his level of arousal because of the intimate connections between the centers of emotion in the brain and the control of his hormonal state. Although the number and vitality of sperm cells may decrease with age, a man may remain fertile throughout his life, able to conceive a child even in his eighties and nineties.

13. The Testis, Epididymis, and Vas Deferens

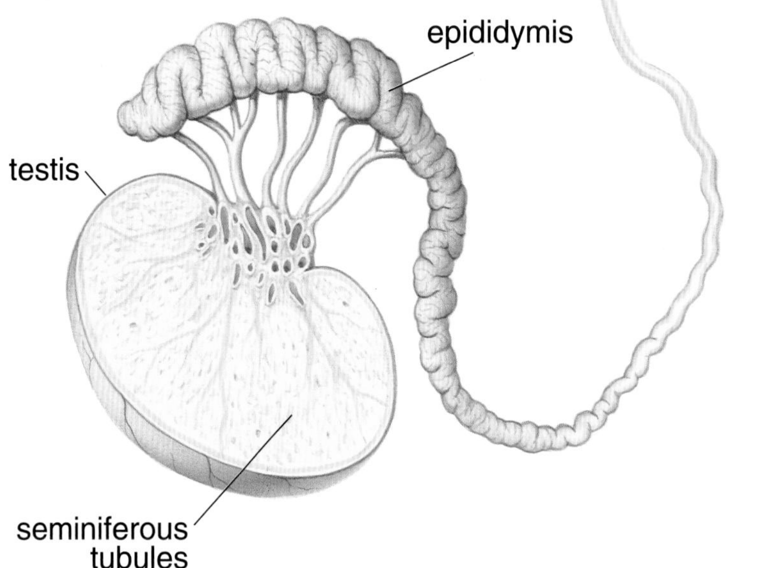

"The hypothalamus and pituitary gland in the brain release hormones that activate sperm production and testosterone release."

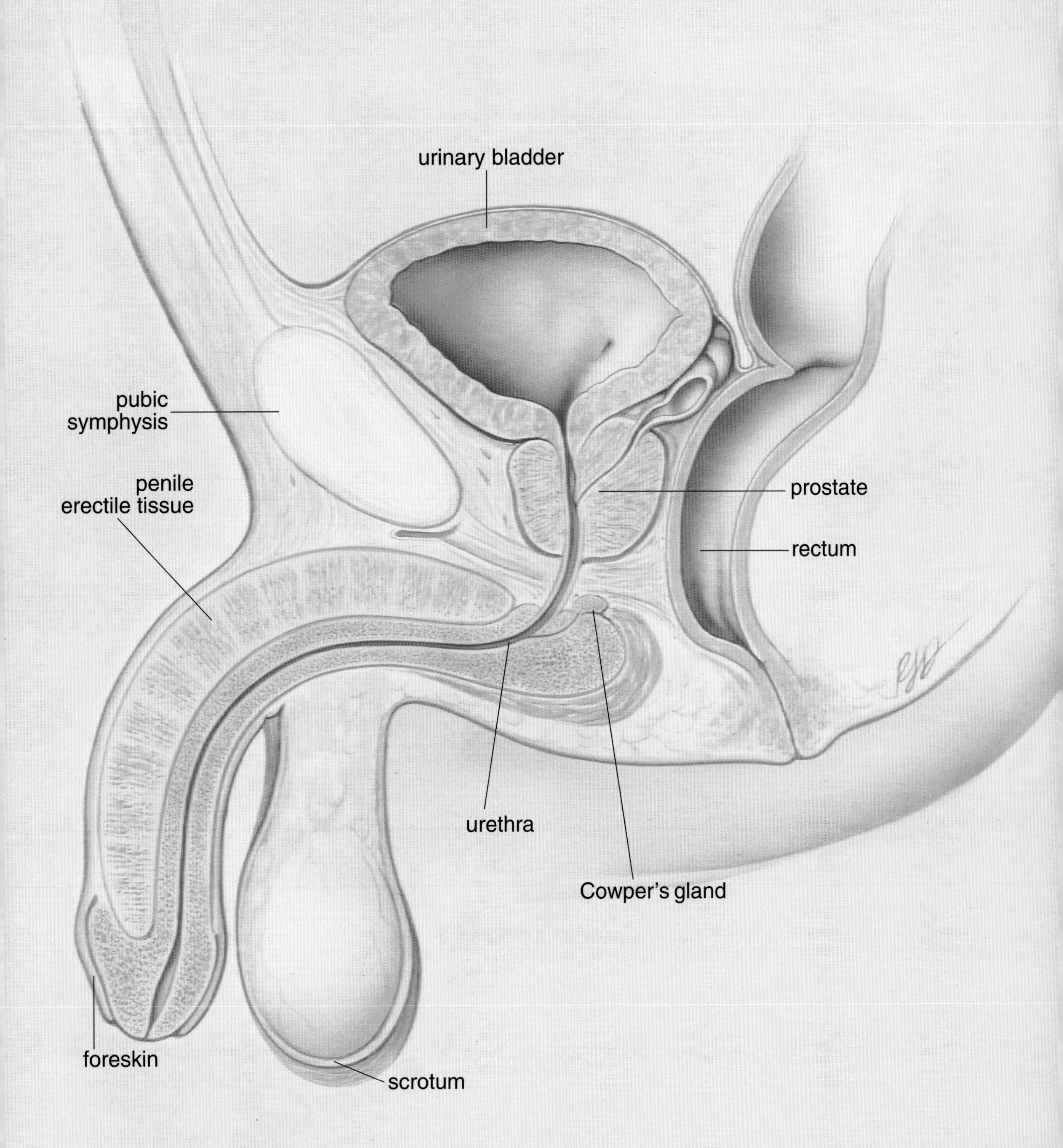
urinary bladder
pubic symphysis
penile erectile tissue
prostate
rectum
urethra
Cowper's gland
foreskin
scrotum

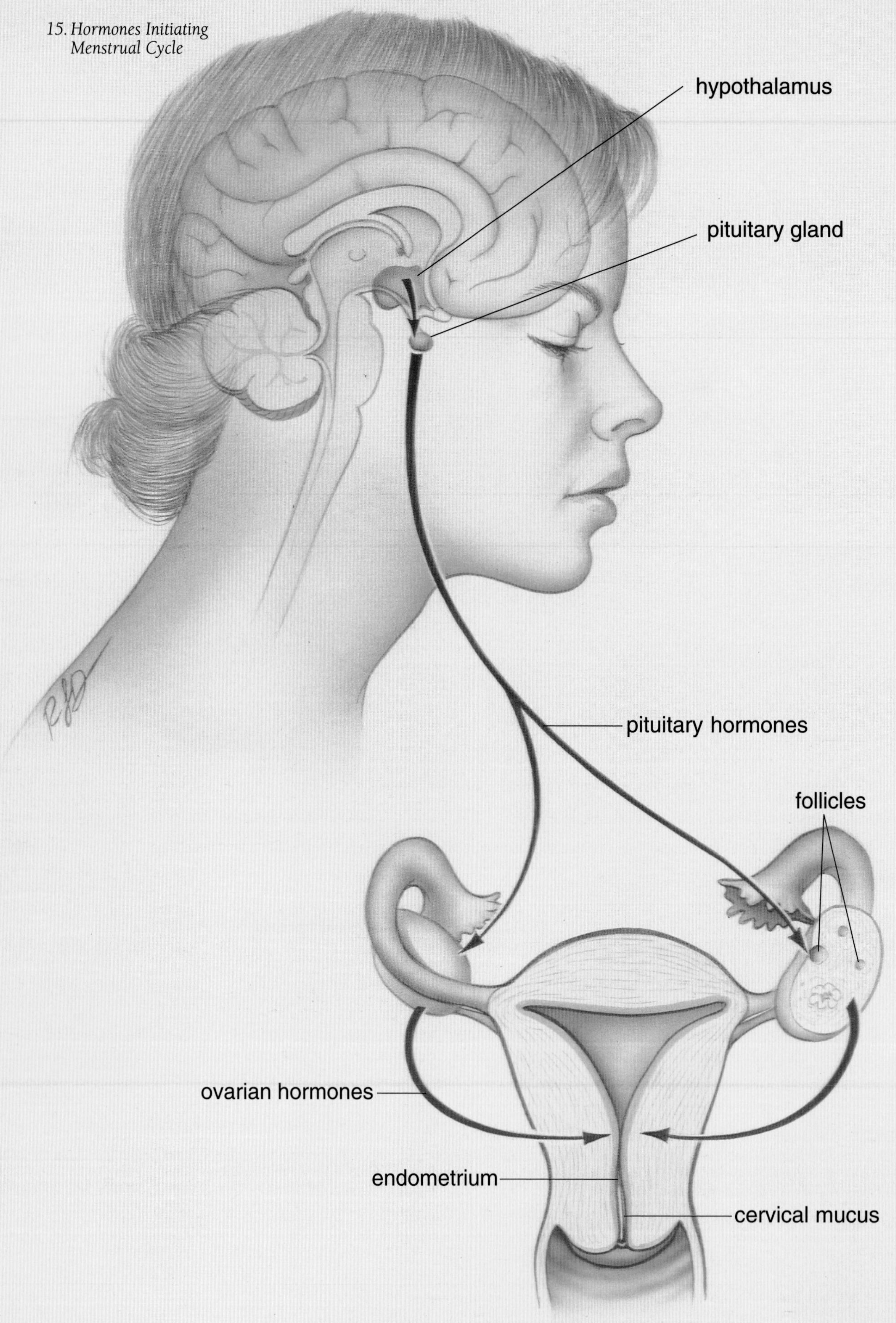
15. Hormones Initiating
Menstrual Cycle
hypothalamus
pituitary gland
pituitary hormones
follicles
ovarian hormones
endometrium
cervical mucus

On the Woman's Side: Development of the Egg

The monthly maturation and release of an egg from the ovary results from a highly synchronized set of events in the brain, the pituitary gland, the ovary, and the uterus. Every month between the onset of periods at the menarche and the end of periods at menopause, a woman goes through a cycle of hormonal and ovarian changes that culminates in ovulation, or egg release. Sometimes the egg joins a sperm resulting in a pregnancy. If not, the woman has a menstrual period and the cycle begins again.

EVENTS IN THE BRAIN

The first step takes place in the brain. A gonadotropin-releasing hormone is discharged from the hypothalamus in the brain. Scientists do not know what triggers the hypothalamus to produce this hormone, although such brain chemicals as dopamine and epinephrine seem to play a part. Unsurprisingly, stress levels, medications that affect the brain, or emotional factors in a woman's life can affect the reproductive cycle.

The gonadotropin-releasing hormone from the hypothalamus enters the blood circulation that bathes the pituitary gland at the center of the brain. When the pituitary gland senses the gonadotropin-releasing hormone, it releases two of its own hormones into the body's bloodstream: luteinizing hormone and follicle-stimulating hormone. These two chemicals travel in the circulatory system to the ovaries where special sensors, or receptors, recognize them.

EVENTS IN THE OVARIES

At the beginning of the cycle, called the follicular phase, these hormones encourage growth of around twenty follicles, each containing an egg, within the ovaries. In a process still mysterious to scientists, one of the developing follicles is chosen to mature. The other follicles collapse within six days, and the chosen follicle, with its egg at its center, enlarges and develops a support system of blood circulation and nutrients. Follicle-stimulating hormone also commands the ovarian follicle to produce the

16. Ovary (in section) with Developing Follicles

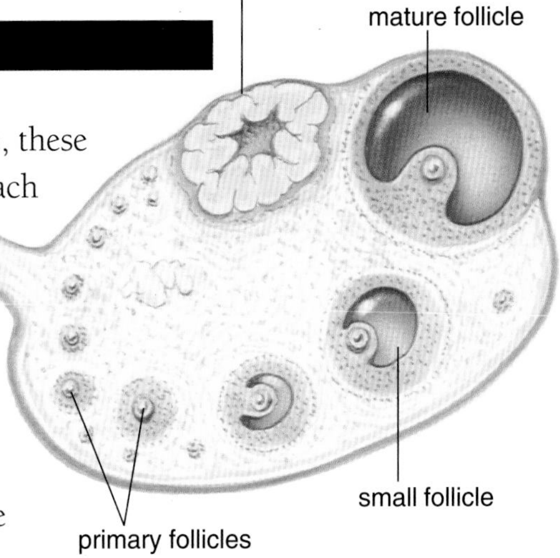

hormone estrogen. When the estrogen level in the blood builds up, it sends a message to the brain and the pituitary to stop releasing the gonadotropin-releasing hormones. These hormones keep one another in a delicate balance through a process called feedback inhibition, in which one hormone leads to the production of a second, and the second, in turn, turns off the production of the first.

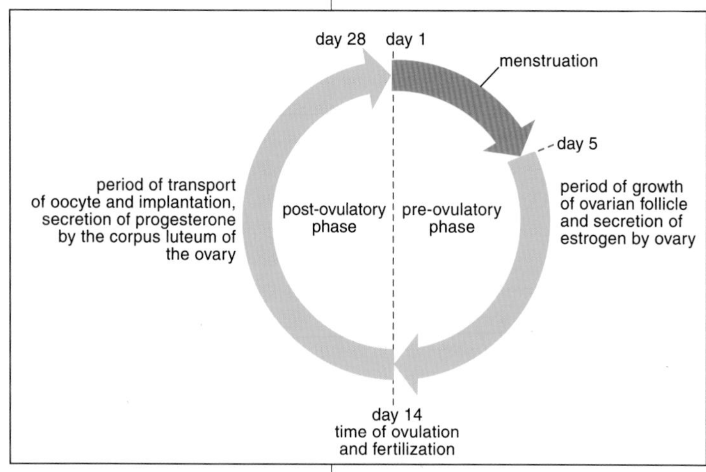

17. Female Reproductive Cycle Diagram

Events in the Uterus

The rising levels of estrogen circulate to the uterus. There, estrogen causes the endometrium, or lining of the uterus, to become more luxurious. The blood supply thickens and the tissue layer deepens, preparing the womb for a potential pregnancy. This phase of the cycle is called the proliferative phase of the endometrium.

The Process of Ovulation

When the follicle is ready to release its egg, it suddenly increases its production of estrogen. The estrogen level in the bloodstream shoots up very dramatically, most of it coming from the chosen follicle. This surge in estrogen triggers an equally dramatic rise in luteinizing hormone and follicle-stimulating hormone. The sudden surge in the pituitary's luteinizing hormone, in a dizzy course of events, turns off estrogen production and turns on the production and release of progesterone, another female sex hormone made in the ovary. Progesterone, together with the luteinizing hormone and follicle-stimulating hormone, precipitates the egg's release.

The egg explodes from the follicle. It is caught by the funnel-shaped end of the Fallopian tube and squeezed down the length of the tube into the chamber of the womb. Once the egg leaves the follicle, the luteal phase begins.

The follicle becomes the corpus luteum, releasing high levels of progesterone. Meanwhile, the rise in the level of progesterone in the circulatory system brings about the secretory phase in the endometrium, during which the uterine lining secretes rich fluids essential for the growth of the fertilized egg.

Alas, this month the egg does not find a sperm cell in the Fallopian tube. If sexual intercourse has not taken place within a few days of ovulation, there will be no union of egg and sperm and no new pregnancy to begin in the womb. Instead, the corpus luteum shrinks to become the corpus albicans and stops producing progesterone. In the absence of estrogen and progesterone, the endometrium loses its bloom. The rich lining of blood and nutrient fluids separate from the walls of the uterus.

For about four or five days, this blood and fluid escape from the uterus through the cervix, causing the woman's period to begin. But already, the next cycle is beginning. During the menstrual period levels of follicle-stimulating hormone climb stimulating next month's follicles to swell in the ovary.

18. Ovulation

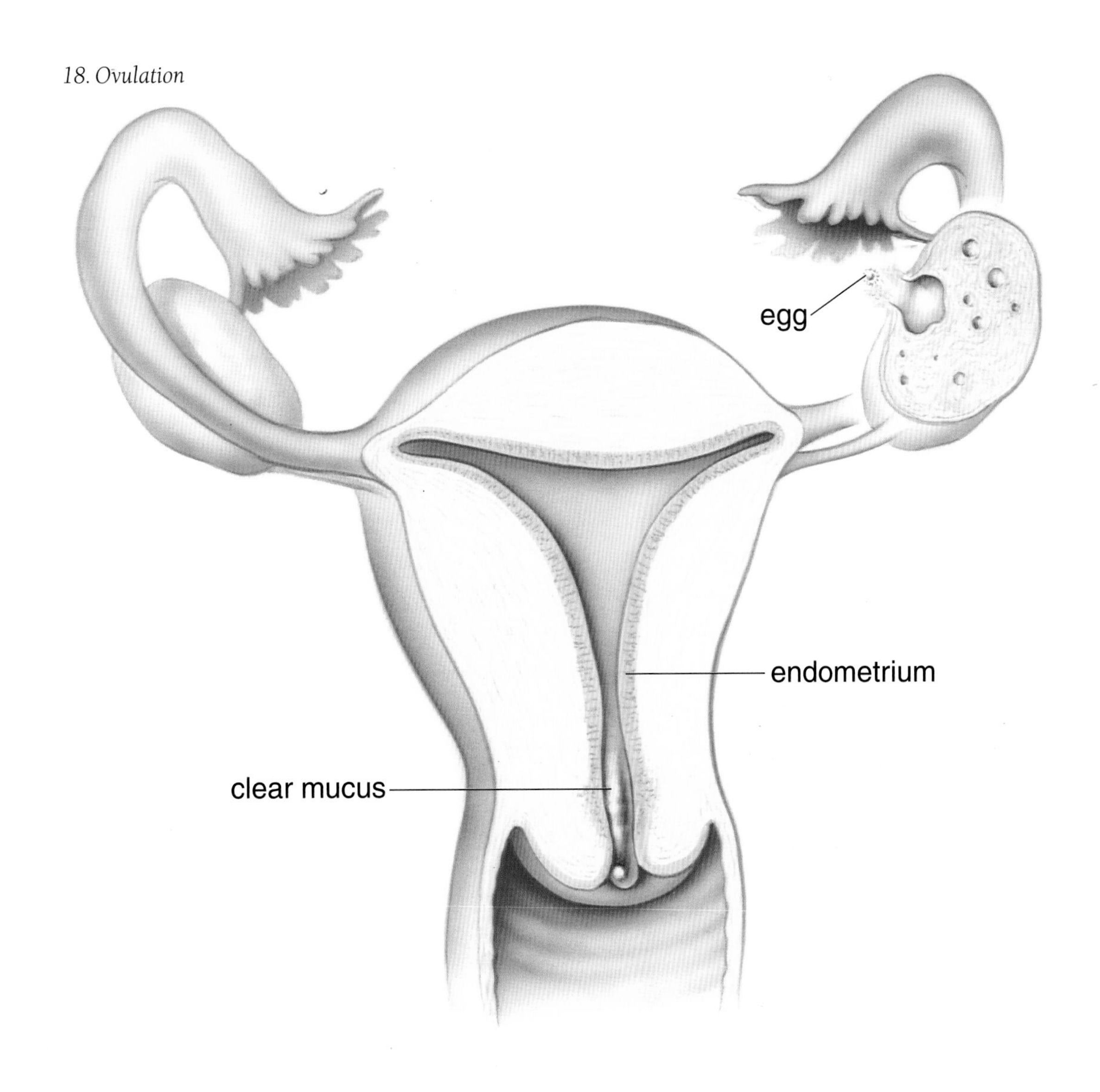

19. Endometrial and Cervical Changes Following Ovulation

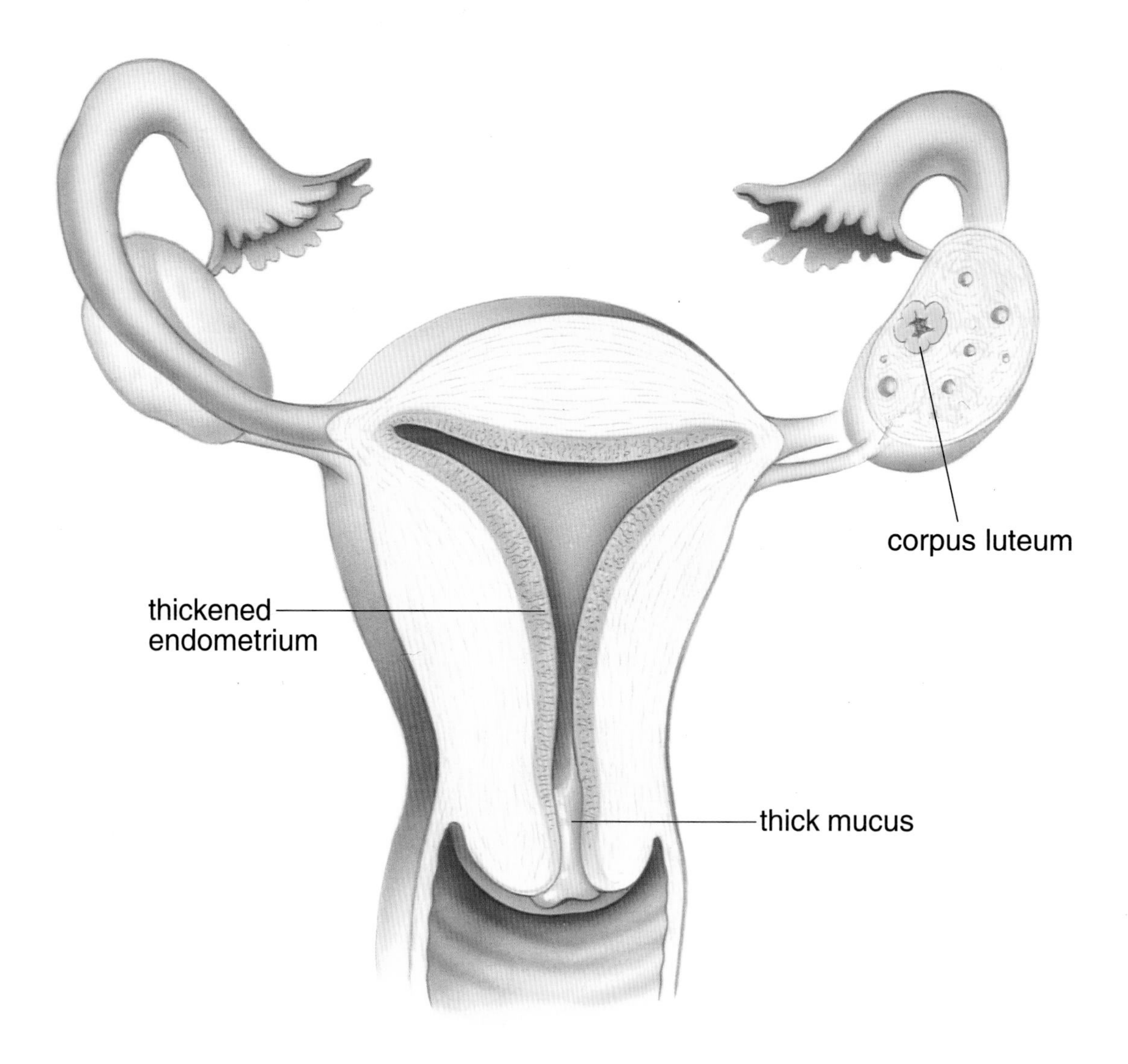

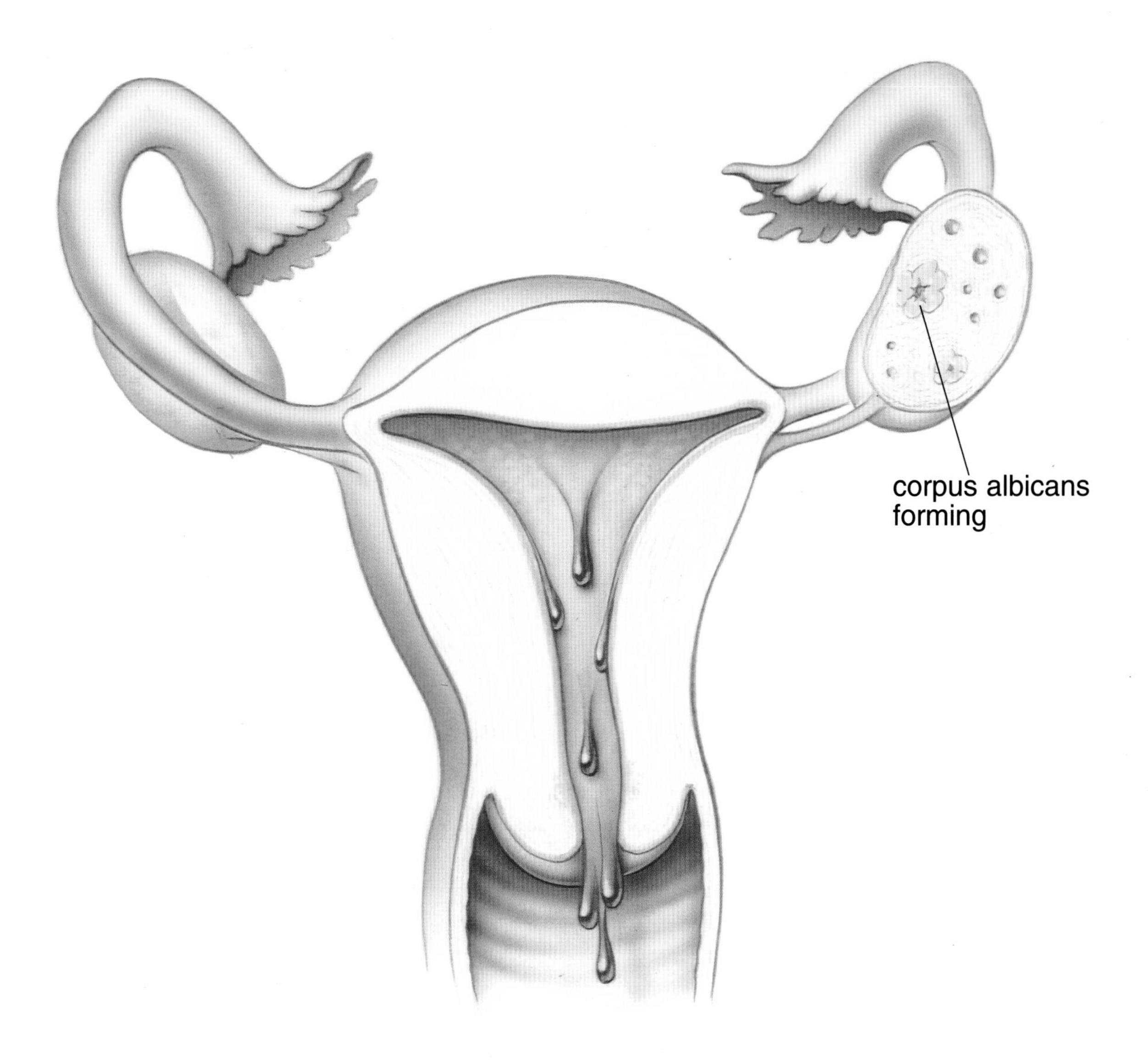
corpus albicans
forming

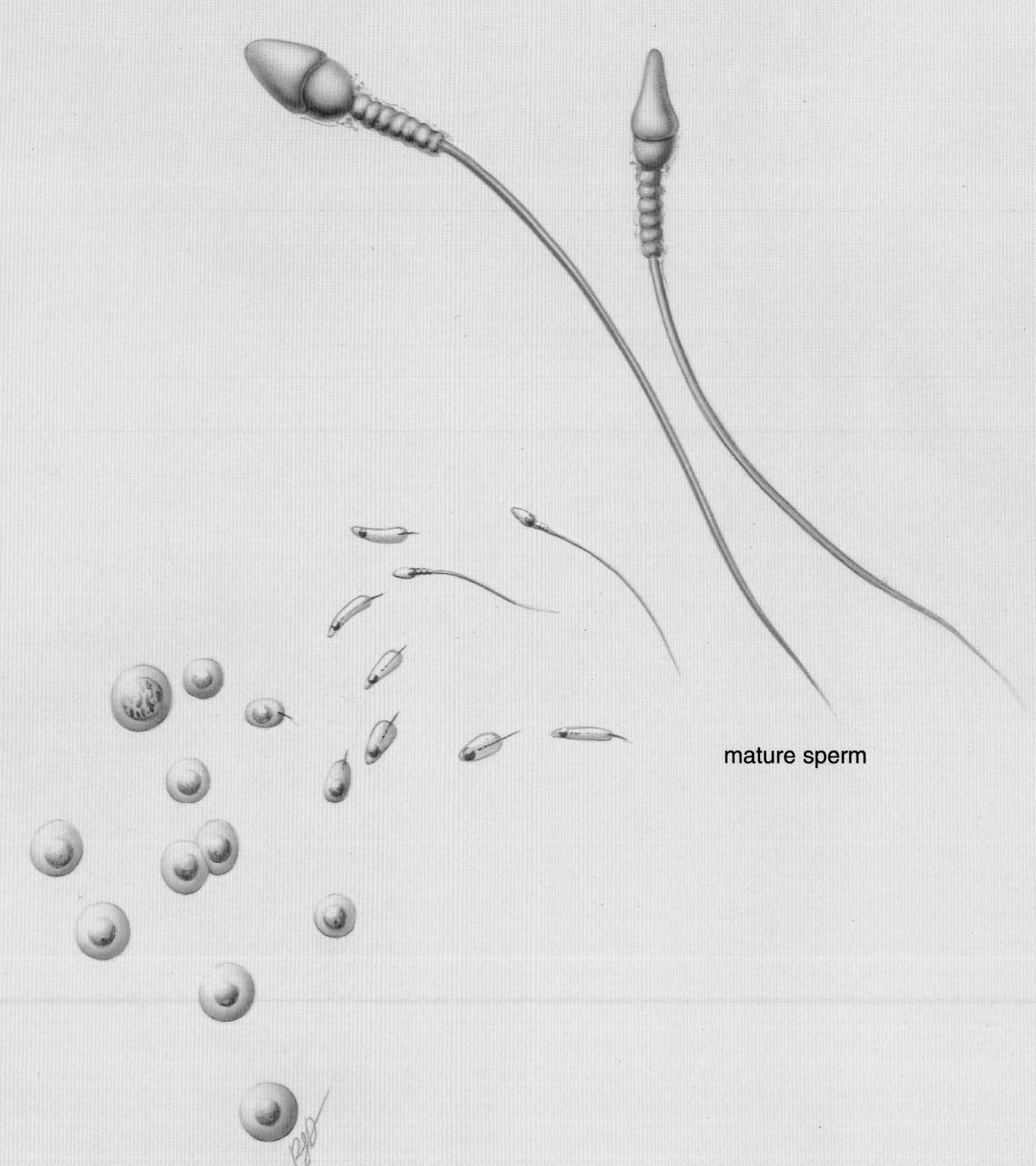

21. Development of the Sperm (much enlarged)

On the Man's Side: Development of the Sperm

From the onset of puberty throughout life, mature sperm cells are continuously produced in the man–millions of them a day. Instead of the monthly cycle of reproduction found in the woman, the man's reproductive cells are constantly and regularly maturing. Groups of sperm mature in waves so that, although it takes 73 days for full development of a sperm cell, there are always plenty of full-grown sperm at any time.

SPERM CELL GROWTH

Deep inside the testes, in the walls of the tightly coiled seminiferous tubules, cells called spermatogonia divide in specialized ways to become spermatocytes. These spermatocytes mature into the spermatids which are eventually released into the tubule's inner open space where they become fully developed spermatozoa, ready, when expelled during an ejaculation, to fertilize an egg.

Sperm cells are unique among human cells. They are almost naked DNA. The only cellular structures besides their clumps of chromosomes are a specialized cap called an acrosome that allows the sperm to penetrate the mother's egg, a neck that produces energy and works like the battery of the sperm, and a tail that allows the sperm to swim very fast. Hundreds of millions of sperm cells are present in the semen of one ejaculation. Scientists have no idea why so many sperm cells are produced, but certainly the healthiest sperms are most successful in reaching the egg for fertilization.

"Hundreds of millions of sperm cells are present in the semen of one ejaculation."

22. Hormones from the Brain and Pituitary Gland Activate Sperm Production and Testosterone Release

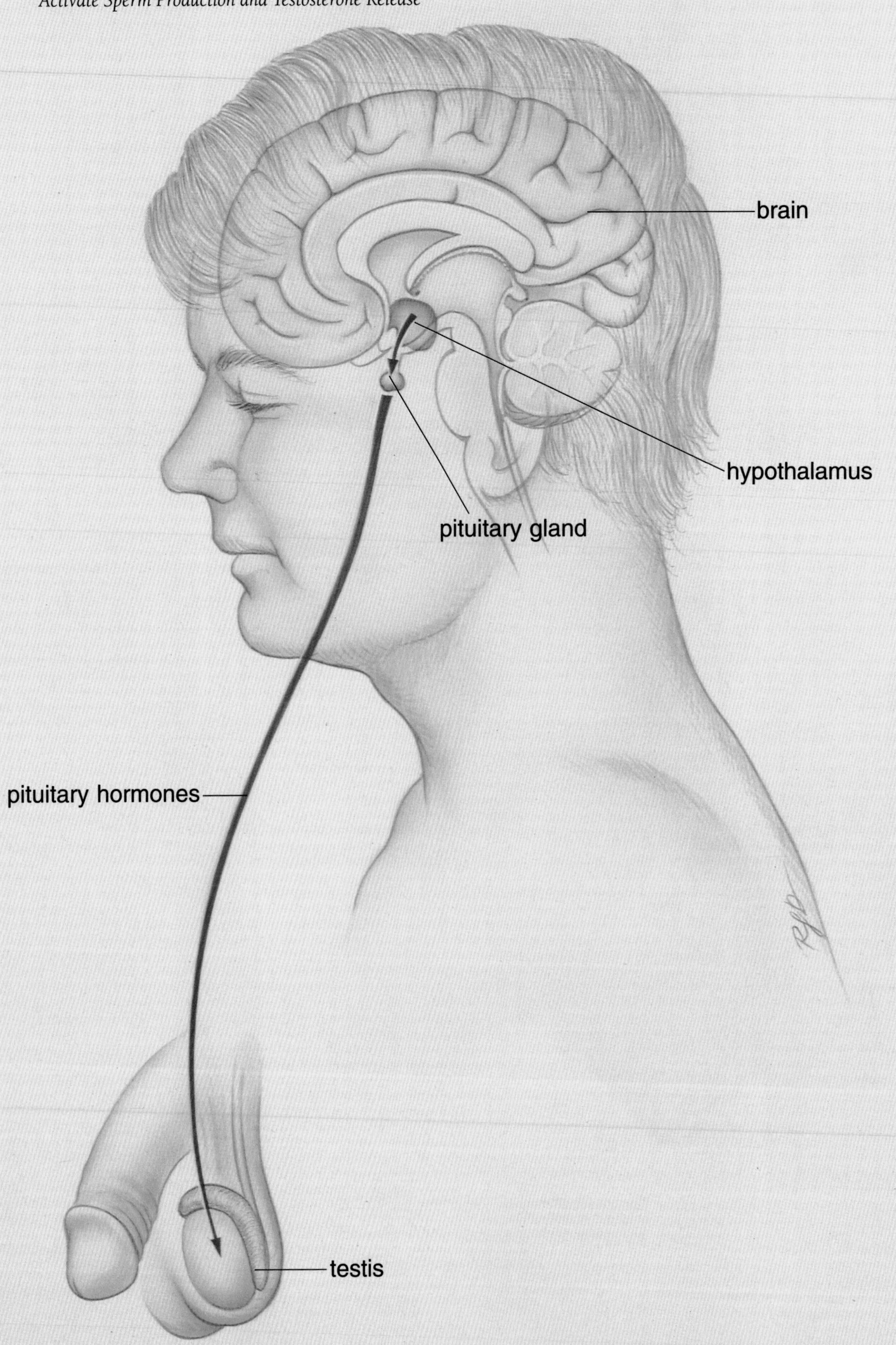

Events in the Brain

Although men and women differ enormously in the number of reproductive cells produced and the timing of their release, both sexes require the same hormonal messages from the hypothalamus and the pituitary gland for reproductive events to take place. As in the woman, gonadotropin-releasing hormone is produced in the man's hypothalamus in the center of the brain and circulates to the pituitary gland. There, the gonadotropin-releasing hormone causes the production and release of the same two hormones described in women–follicle-stimulating hormone and luteinizing hormone. Years ago, biologists gave these hormones different names when they were found in men instead of women, but, in fact, they are biochemically identical. Today we use the same names whether found in a woman or a man, even though their names refer to events that occur in the woman's body.

> *"Created from cholesterol, testosterone is also responsible for the secondary sex characteristics of a man, like beard growth, penile growth, deepening of the voice, and growth of the Adam's apple."*

Events in the Testes

When luteinizing hormone and follicle-stimulating hormone are carried to the testes, they promote sperm maturation in the seminiferous tubules and cause special cells called Leydig cells to produce testosterone and related male sex hormones. In turn, testosterone helps the sperm to mature. Created from cholesterol, testosterone is also responsible for the secondary sex characteristics of a man, such as beard growth, penile growth, deepening of the voice, and growth of the Adam's apple. In addition, testosterone and the other male hormones called androgens encourage libido and sexual performance. If the woman's role in reproduction is to produce the egg and nurture and protect the developing child throughout pregnancy and delivery, the man's role is to produce the sperm and to deposit it as close to the woman's egg as he can. Thus, his entire reproductive apparatus is geared toward interest in and success in intercourse.

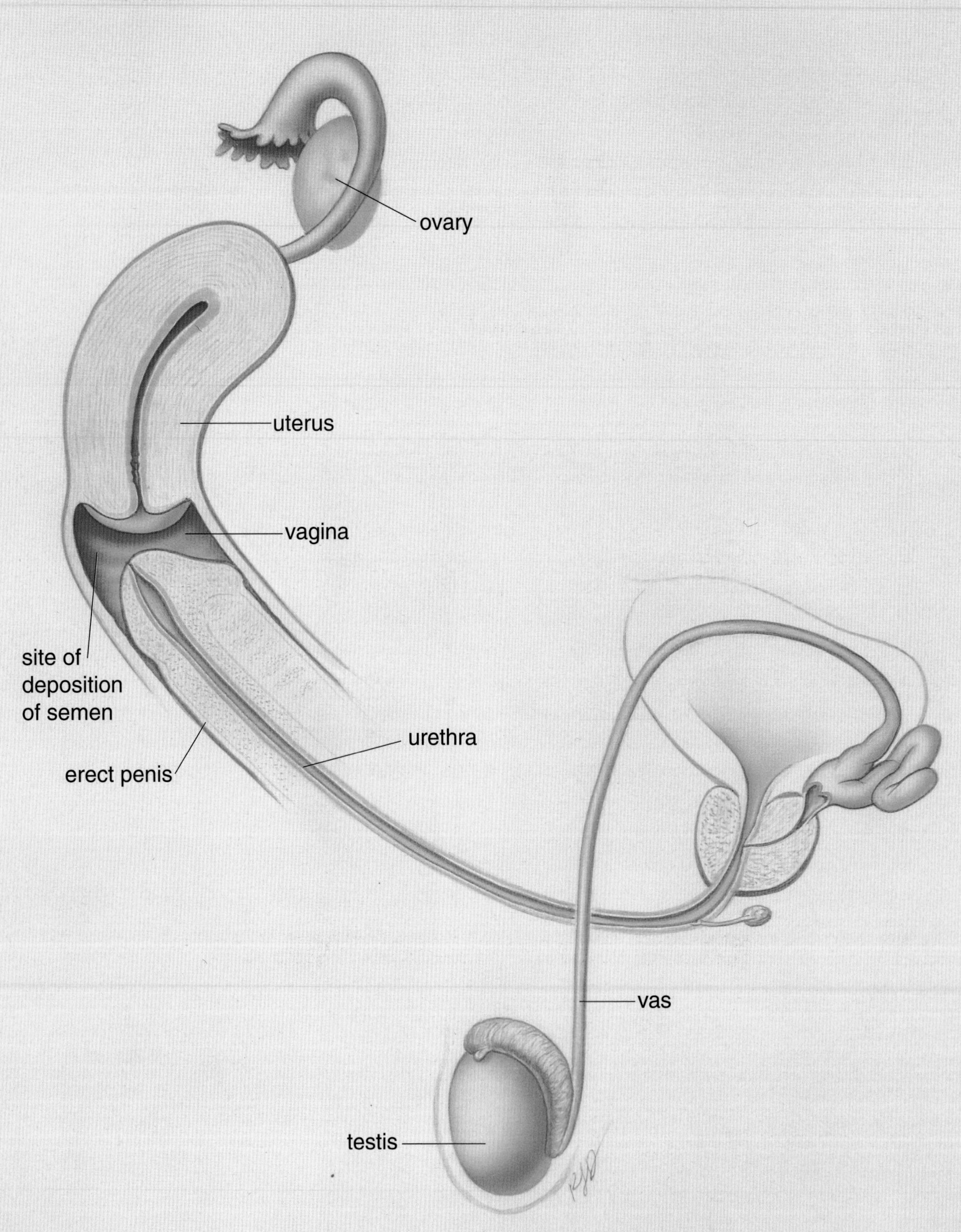
ovary
uterus
vagina
site of
deposition
of semen
urethra
erect penis
vas
testis

Man and Woman: Sexual Intercourse

Both the female hormone estrogen and the male hormone testosterone awaken sexual desire and prepare the body for erotic pleasure and intercourse. Through somewhat mysterious processes in the brain, sexual interest is aroused by visual and tactile stimuli or even through acts of the imagination. Sexual arousal, in turn, causes specific changes in the man's and the woman's body to allow the marvelously choreographed act of intercourse to take place.

SEXUAL AROUSAL

In the woman, sexual arousal causes enlargement of the clitoris. Secretions from Bartholin's and Skene's glands lubricate the vagina, preparing the woman to accept the penis into her vagina. The man's body changes in more dramatic ways when sexually aroused. Nerve impulses to the penis cause its blood circulation to increase many-fold. The penis doubles in size, becoming stiff and erect. At the same time, different sets of nerve impulses command the epididymis, the vas deferens, and the sexual glands to contract, releasing their fluids into the urethra in the process of emission.

"Sexual arousal causes specific changes in the man's and the woman's body to allow the marvelously choreographed act of intercourse to take place."

Sexual arousal ordinarily leads first to foreplay, during which the entire bodies of the man and woman become erotically stimulated. The breasts and nipples, the earlobes, the lips, the back of the neck, and the inside of the thighs are all highly sensitive areas where men and women can give one another pleasure. Although there are countless sexual behaviors known, penile penetration into the vagina (or deposition of the semen into the vagina) is the only sexual act that can lead to reproduction.

COITUS

Once the penis is erect and the vagina well lubricated, the man is able to insert his penis into the woman in the act called coitus. The glans of the penis becomes highly sensitive when the penis is erect, and as it is massaged by penetration, the man's arousal is heightened. At the peak of sexual pleasure, the man experiences orgasm, during which the muscles of the penis undergo rapid and forceful contractions. These contractions force the fluids containing the sperm out of the penis and into the woman's vagina, in the act of ejaculation. Meanwhile, the woman too may experience orgasm, possibly both at the clitoris and within the vagina, although female orgasm is not necessary for a pregnancy to occur. Incidentally, biologists believe that humans are the only mammal species in which the female experiences orgasm. Chemicals called prostaglandins in the man's ejaculate act directly on the muscle of the woman's uterus to cause further contractions, helping to direct sperm into the uterus.

"Of all the sperm deposited in the vagina, less than 200 will swim into the caverns of the uterus and toward the Fallopian tube where, if ovulation has just occurred, the egg waits."

The cervical mucus changes over the course of the woman's menstrual cycle. At the middle of her cycle, around the time of ovulation, the cervical mucus becomes fluid and plentiful. It is less acidic than at other times in the cycle and therefore easier for sperm to cross. Although many of the millions of sperm do not pass through the cervical mucus, the strongest ones do. These few will escape from the acidity of the vagina, where no sperm can survive for long, and swim up through the cervical mucus into the entrance to the uterus. Of all the sperm deposited in the vagina, less than 200 will swim into the caverns of the uterus and toward the Fallopian tube where, if ovulation has just occurred, the egg waits.

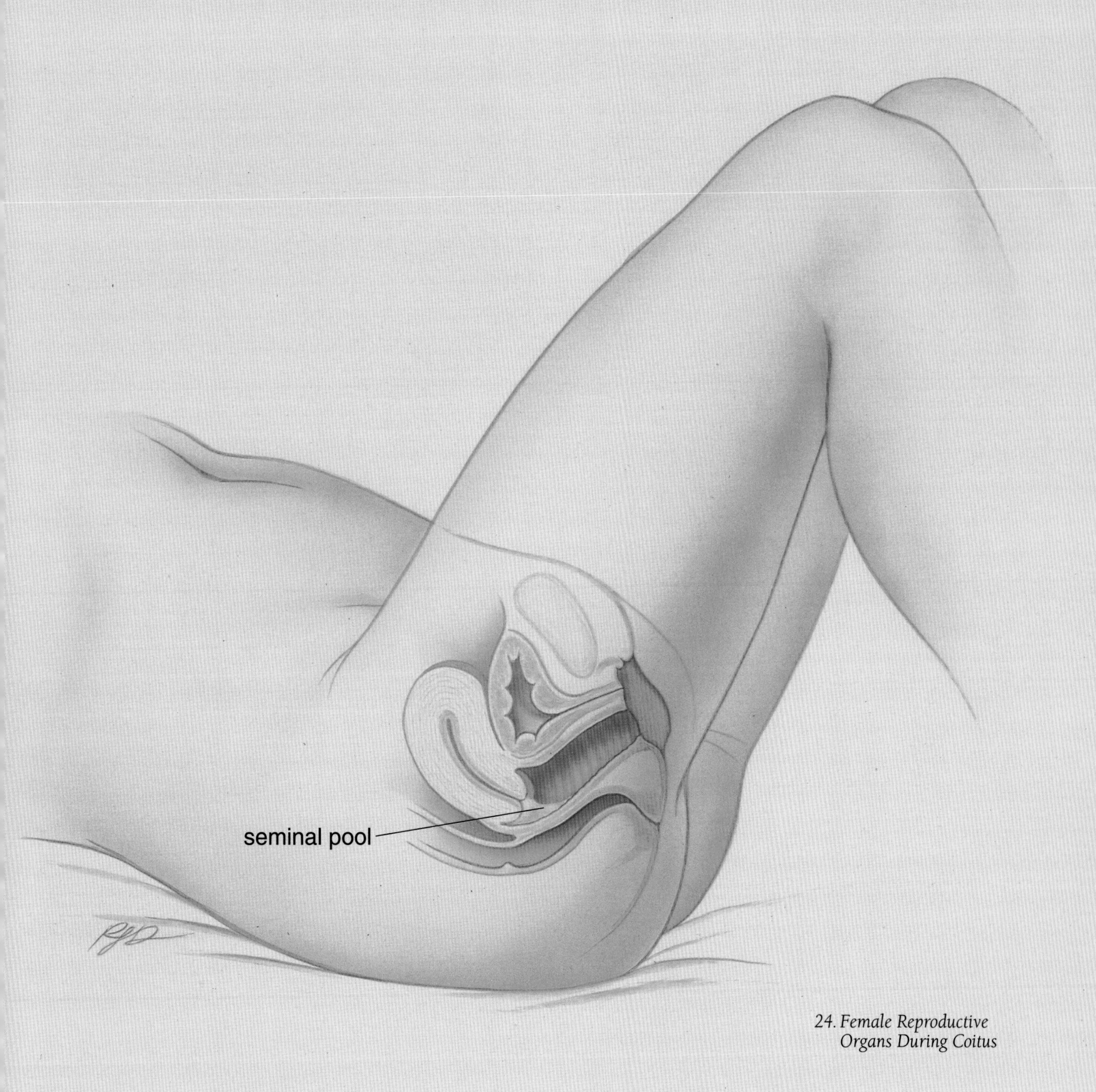

24. Female Reproductive Organs During Coitus

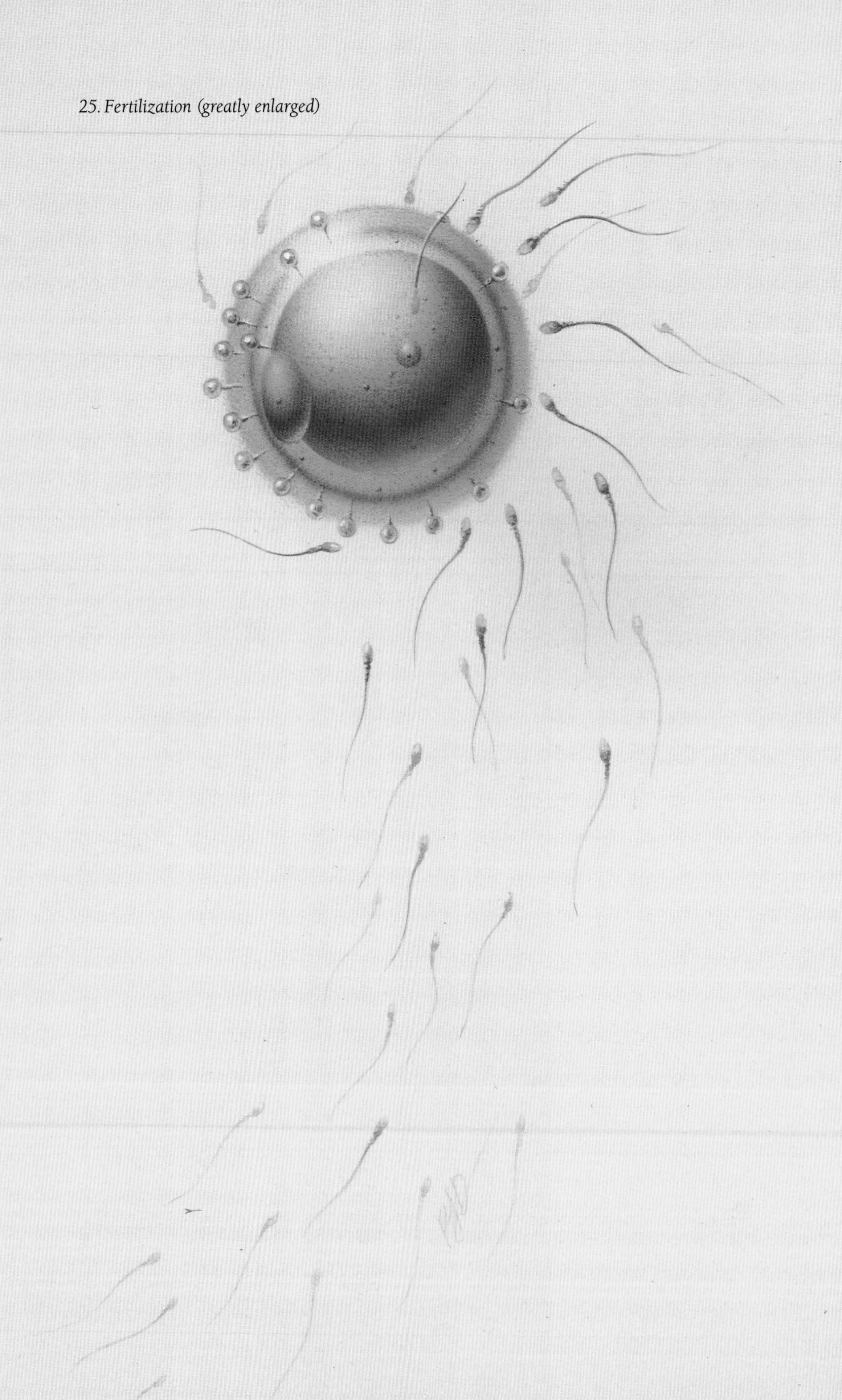

25. Fertilization (greatly enlarged)

Man and Woman: Fertilization and Implantation

The egg has developed within the ovary of the woman, and the sperm has developed within the testicle of the man. In the act of sexual intercourse or through artificial insemination, the man's sperm is brought within the vagina of the woman. This chapter will describe the joining of the egg and the sperm in the step called fertilization. One sperm cell enters the egg, causing the genes of the man to combine with the genes of the woman. A few days after fertilization, the fertilized egg becomes implanted in the lining of the uterus where it will become the embryo, the fetus, and finally the baby.

FERTILIZATION

The sperm cells that cross through the cervical mucus enter the uterus and congregate at the openings of the Fallopian tubes or sink into the crevices of the cervix. There they may stay for a few days, quiescently, until ovulation occurs and sends a message that they are welcome to enter the tubes. As the sperm cells travel through the woman's reproductive tract, they undergo another change, called capacitation, that helps them to fertilize an egg.

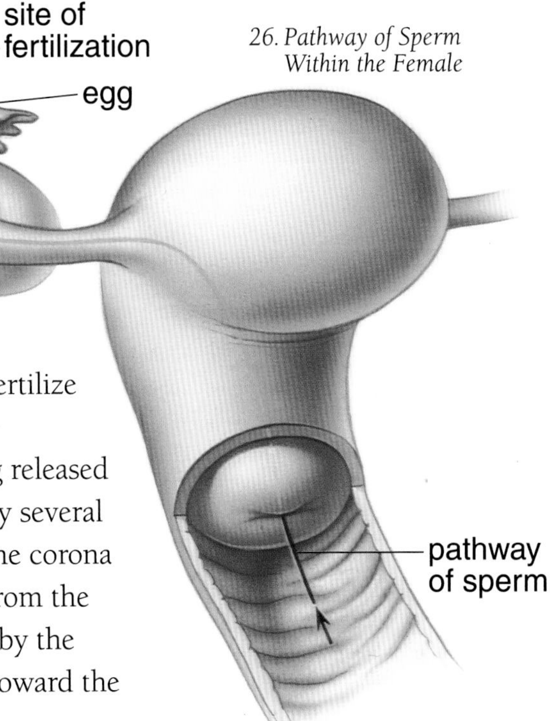

26. Pathway of Sperm Within the Female

Meanwhile, if ovulation is occurring, the egg is being released from the ovary. Upon ovulation, the egg is surrounded by several layers of protective cells: first, the zona pellucida, then the corona radiata, and finally, the cumulus oophorus. Once freed from the ovary, the egg with its gelatinous coverings is picked up by the contracting fimbriae of the Fallopian tube and directed toward the uterus.

Fertilization occurs within minutes to up to thirty-six hours after ovulation. Sperm may wait within the uterus for the ovulated egg for two to three days, and the egg survives after ovulation for about 36 hours. Therefore, as a general guideline, fertilization is possible if intercourse occurs from 72 hours before ovulation to 36 hours after ovulation. If an egg does not meet a sperm within 36 hours of its release from the ovary, it degenerates and the woman must wait until her next cycle if she desires a pregnancy.

The egg and the sperm make an odd couple. At a diameter of around a tenth of a millimeter, the egg is hundreds of times larger than the sperm. Regal in its protective coatings, the egg is borne on its travels by the beating cilia of the Fallopian tube while the naked sperm swims strenuously against the current to reach its prize. Despite their outward differences, these two were made for each other. The egg has particular sites on its surface called receptors that recognize the sperm and bind to it. One sperm out of the hundreds that have survived the trip to the Fallopian tube is somehow fated to fertilize the egg. This sperm attaches to the egg, sheds its cap, or acrosome, and releases enzymes that dissolve the outer coverings of the egg. In about three hours, the entire sperm enters the egg. Simultaneously, changes occur in the egg as soon as the sperm has entered it, rearranging the zona pellucida so that no other sperm can gain entrance. The egg is now said to be fertilized, having the potential to develop into a new baby.

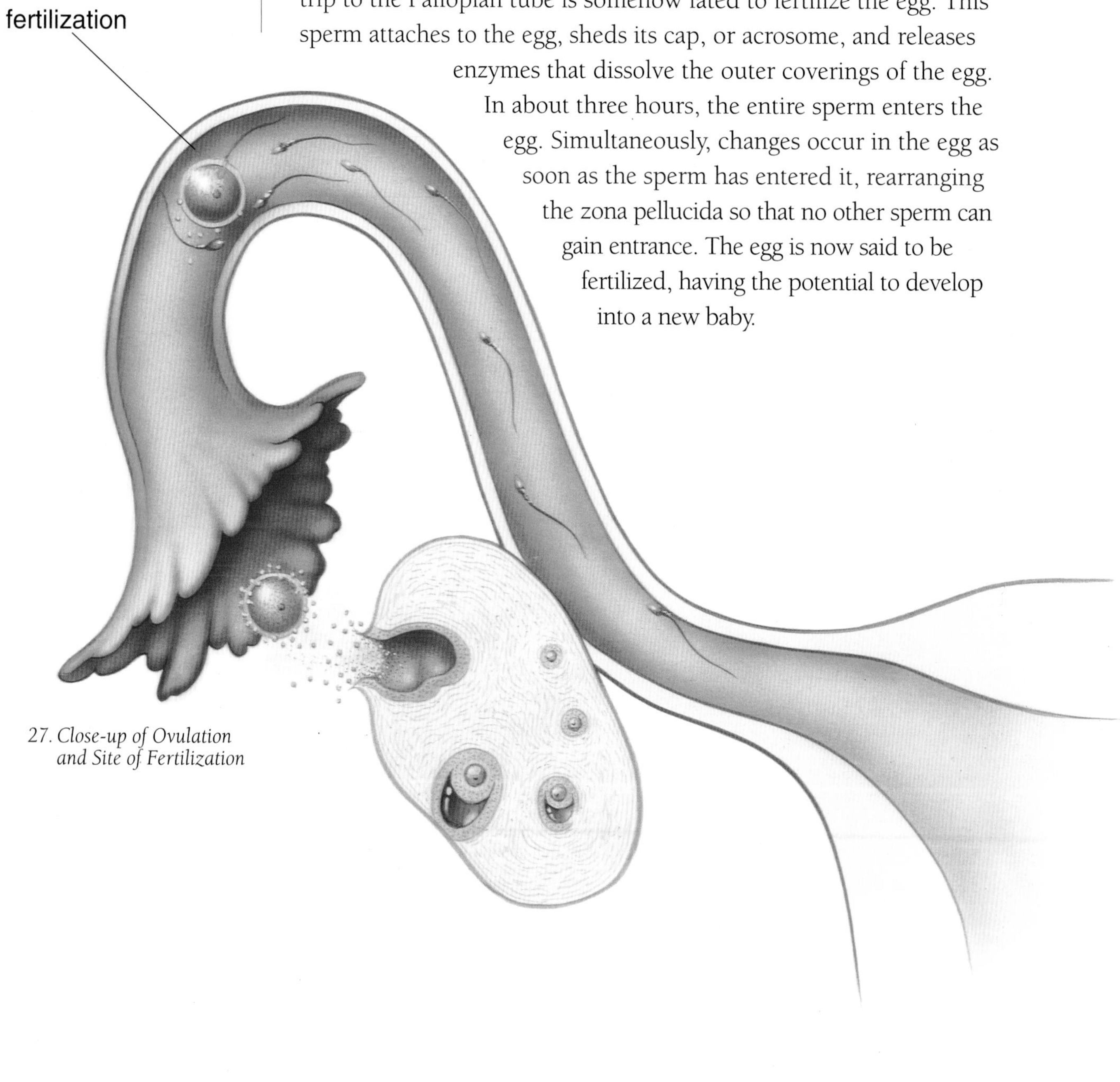

fertilization

27. Close-up of Ovulation and Site of Fertilization

GENES AND BIOLOGICAL TRAITS

All the cells in a person's body, with two exceptions, contain 46 chromosomes arranged in 23 pairs, one member of each pair originating from the person's mother and the other member of the pair originating from the father. Each chromosome contains thousands and thousands of genes, and each gene is made up of long spirals of DNA. The DNA's genetic code determines all our biological characteristics, like eye color, height, and presence or absence of inherited diseases. The exceptions to the rule of 46 are the egg and the sperm. The sperm cell and the egg cell have only 23 chromosomes because of the way the sperm and egg cells divide during their maturation. When a sperm cell fertilizes an egg cell, the sperm's 23 chromosomes pair up with the egg's 23 chromosomes to produce the normal number of 46 chromosomes.

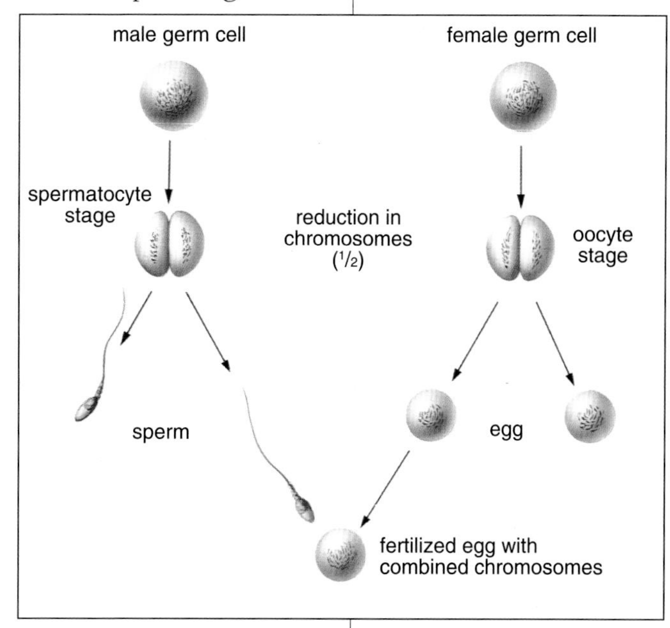

28. Uniting of Chromosomes from Male and Female

The genetic material of the egg and the sperm merge, combining the hereditary traits from the woman and the man to determine future biological characteristics of the potential child. Although most biological features are determined by both the mother's and the father's genes, it is the father's sperm alone that determines the sex of the baby. Each child gets two sex chromosomes, one from the mother and one from the father. There are only two kinds of sex chromosomes, Xs and Ys. All eggs contain X chromosomes, so the mother can only give her child an X chromosome. Half the sperm a man makes contain X chromosomes and half contain Y chromosomes. If the father's sperm cell brings an X chromosome, the baby will be a girl, biologically called XX. If the father gives a sperm with a Y chromosome, the baby will be a boy–an XY.

In the rare instance where two eggs are released by the ovary at the same time and each egg is fertilized by a sperm, two pregnancies would occur. Born at the same time, but not identical, because they develop from different combinations of egg and sperm the babies would be fraternal twins.

IMPLANTATION

The fertilized egg divides several times while traveling down the Fallopian tube. After three days, the fertilized egg has become a small mulberry-shaped ball of cells called the morula, sometimes only twelve or sixteen cells in all. The morula develops a central cavity and is now a cyst called the blastocyst. The blastocyst burrows into the uterine wall about a week after fertilization. This process is called implantation. The implanted blastocyst releases proteins and hormones, including human chorionic gonadotropin hormone, to signal to the woman's ovary that fertilization has occurred. These hormonal messages tell the corpus luteum in the ovary to continue to produce progesterone and estrogen. Because the levels of estrogen and progesterone do not drop, the woman will not have a menstrual period this cycle. This is the missed period that alerts her that she may be pregnant. Instead, the blood and tissue of her uterine lining will be used to form the placenta.

The fertilized egg enters the uterus as a morula and develops into the blastocyst, which has fifty to sixty cells. The zona pellucida has disappeared by this time. In addition to the material derived from the egg and the sperm, the blastocyst has accumulated fluid and nutrients.

29. Development of the Egg as it Moves Down the Tube and Attaches to Endometrium

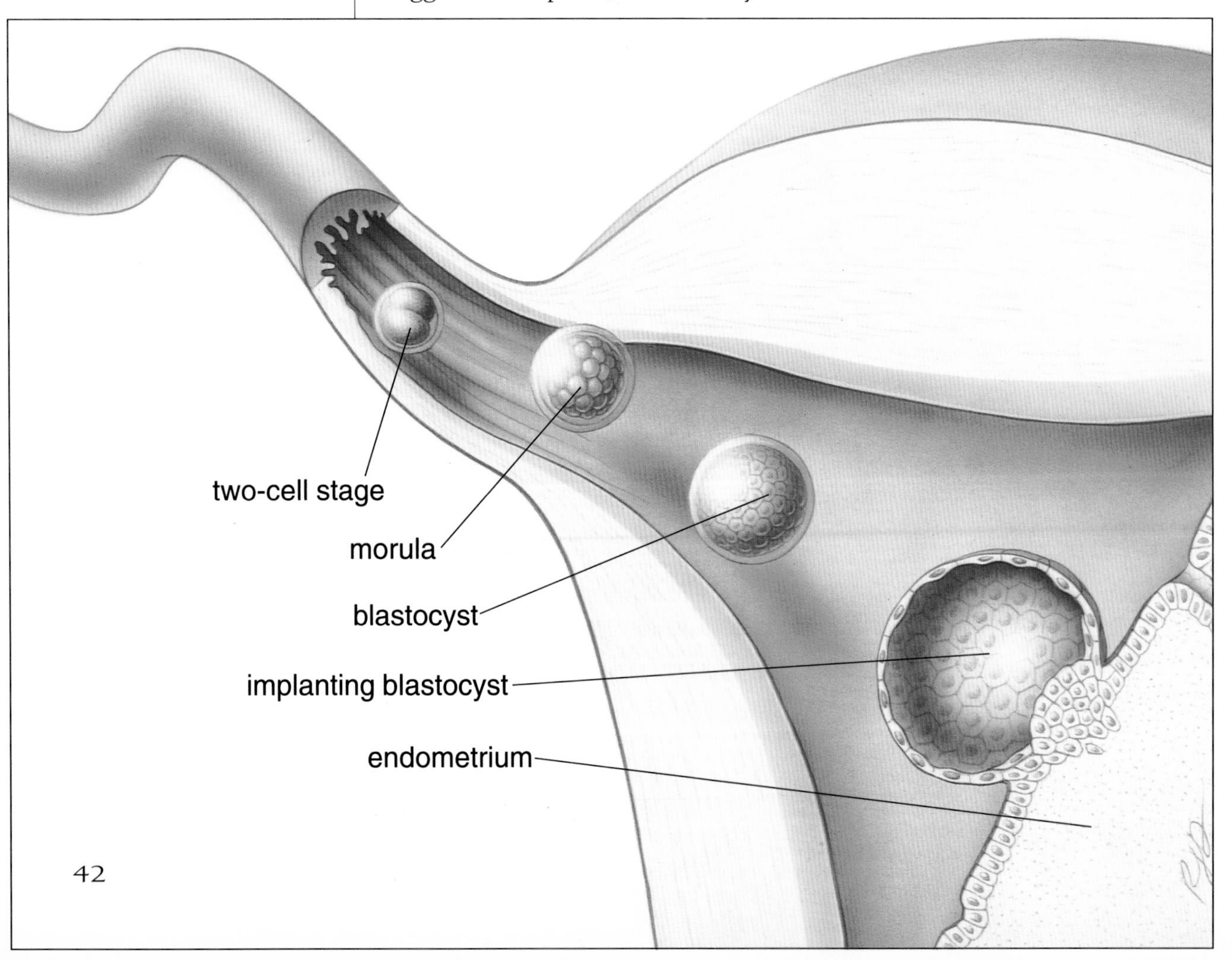

Part of the blastocyst will become the embryo, and the rest, the trophoblast, will contribute to the placenta. Meanwhile, the uterus is preparing to accept the blastocyst, in part as a result of the blastocyst's hormones. At this point in the cycle, immediately after ovulation, the uterine lining is at its peak of luxuriance and secretory lushness.

By six or seven days after ovulation, the blastocyst has attached itself to the inner lining of the womb. The part of the blastocyst deepest within the uterine wall will become the placenta, while immediately above it is found the embryo. The pregnancy has begun. In some cases, the blastocyst separates before attachment and implantation and results in two embryos and, if term is complete, twins. These twins would be identical twins because they developed from the same egg and the same sperm, so all their chromosomes would be the same. At other times, the blastocyst does not enter the uterus but, instead, attaches to the Fallopian tube, the ovary, or another abdominal organ. Such a pregnancy is called an ectopic pregnancy. It cannot become a full-term pregnancy and must be surgically interrupted as it poses a potential grave danger to the woman.

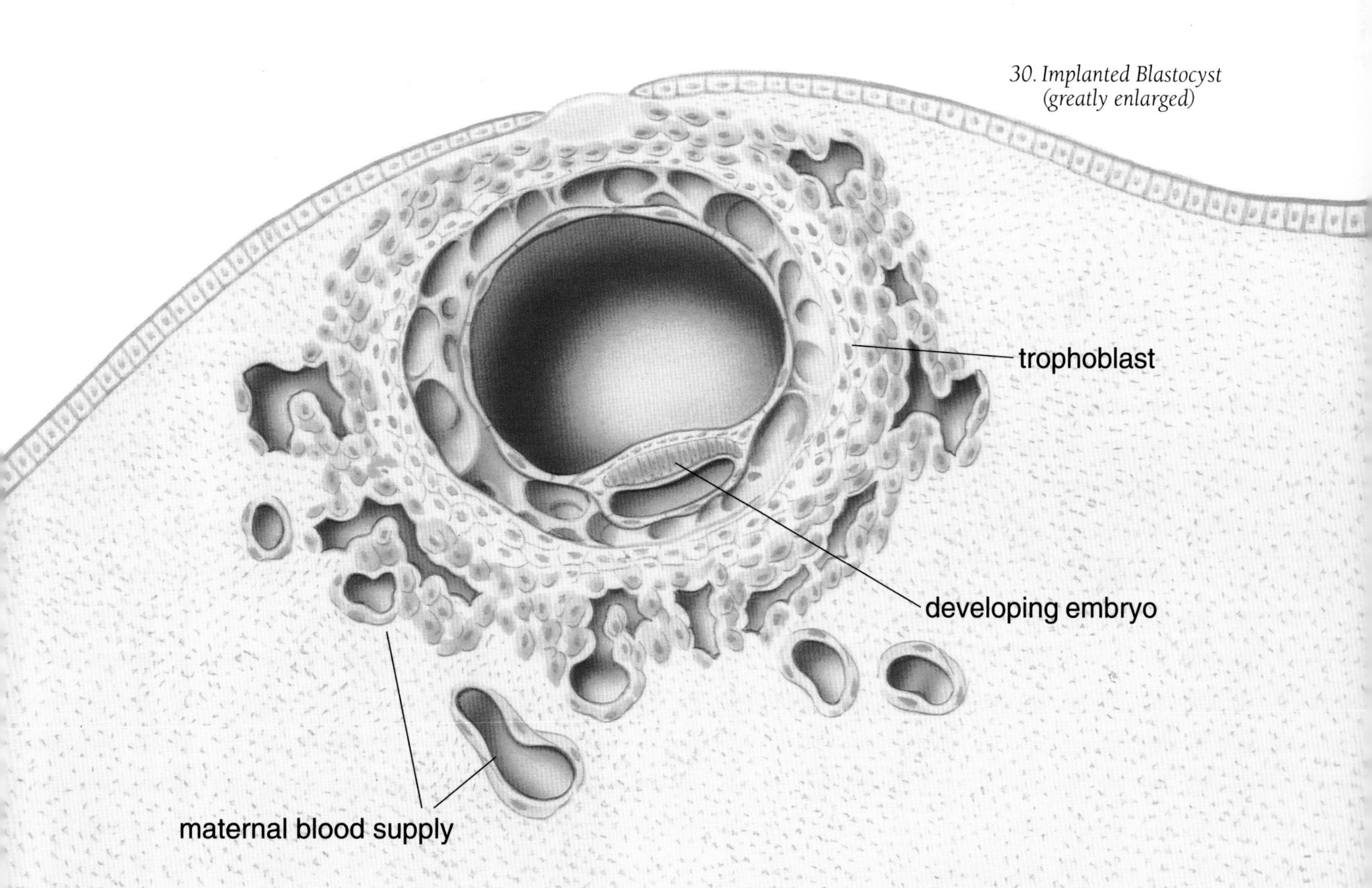

30. Implanted Blastocyst (greatly enlarged)

Confirming the Pregnancy

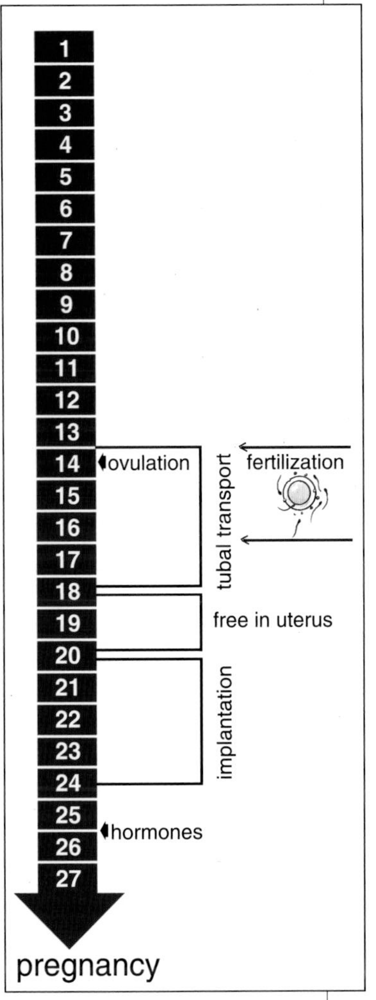

31. Time Sequence From Day 1 of Menstrual Cycle to Pregnancy

Pregnancy can be confirmed by tests done at home or tests done in the doctor's office, although the urine tests done at home are not as accurate as the blood test done by the laboratory. Both urine and blood tests measure the presence of human chorionic gonadotropin, the hormone produced by the blastocyst itself. A definite "yes" about a pregnancy can be given as early as two weeks after fertilization, coinciding with the time that the first missed period is expected. With help from her doctor or partner, the woman will decide whether to continue the pregnancy.

By convention, the pregnancy will be dated from the last menstrual period. The obstetrician will take the first day of the last menstrual period, add seven days to that, and count back three months to calculate the so-called estimated date of confinement (the Victorian term for the seclusion a birthing mother used to endure). This dating actually overestimates the age of the embryo by about two weeks, because fertilization occurs not one week but two weeks after the beginning of the last period and the length of the entire pregnancy is somewhat longer than nine months. This dating scheme can be inaccurate in a woman who was taking oral contraceptives when she became pregnant, or a woman who has unpredictable or irregular periods. Nonetheless, this calculated date is useful in estimating the time of arrival of the new baby. However it is measured, the length of full-term pregnancy is amazingly constant at very close to 266 days or 38 weeks from fertilization or 280 days from the last menstrual period.

Pregnancies are often divided by obstetricians into thirds, or trimesters because particular steps in development or particular problems can be encountered in either the first, second, or third trimester. Obstetricians may also refer to the gestational age of the developing fetus in terms of weeks, as more knowledge is accumulating about very specific events occurring within each week of growth. Accurate dating of the fetus is now easily done with images obtained from an ultrasonogram. Ultrasonograms are images created by the patterns of sound waves when a special microphone is pointed at a part of the body. Because an ultrasono-gram is a relatively safe and painless procedure, it is used by physicians in many areas of medicine.

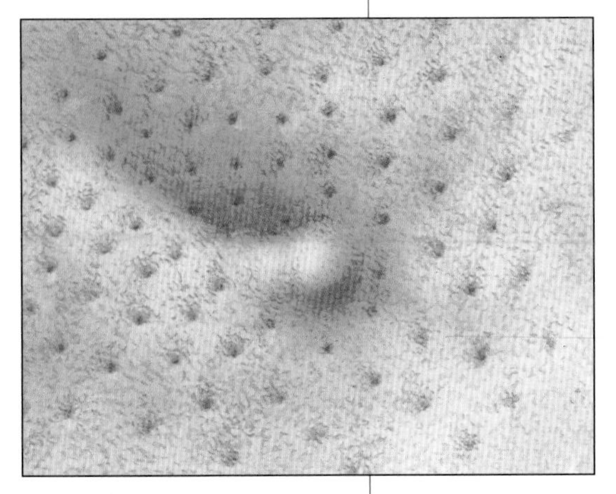

32. Magnified Surface View of Implanted Blastocyst

Mother and Embryo: The Early Pregnancy

Once the blastocyst is implanted in the uterine lining, it is called an embryo. Following the first eight weeks within the uterus (or ten weeks after the last menstrual period), the embryo is called the fetus.

Prenatal Care

On the first visit to the obstetrician or nurse-midwife, the pregnant woman will be examined and pregnancy confirmed with a blood test and pelvic examination. If the woman chooses to continue with the pregnancy, prenatal care will be instituted to attend to the mother and embryo's health, to manage any of the woman's medical problems, and to advise her against such activities as drinking alcohol, smoking cigarettes, using drugs, or taking any medications that may harm the embryo. Prenatal care will make sure that the woman has been vaccinated against such infections as German measles and hepatitis that could disrupt embryonic development and will offer testing for such infections as HIV, syphilis, and gonorrhea that could have grave consequences for woman and child. Throughout the pregnancy, the doctor or nurse will measure uterine size, blood pressure, weight, sugar in the blood, and protein in the urine and will give recommendations for nutrition and vitamins needed to keep mother and child healthy. If a woman has medical illnesses herself, if she has had complicated pregnancies in the past, if she is undernourished, or if she is very young, her pregnancy will be considered a high-risk pregnancy and she will be offered more frequent and more detailed medical check-ups.

33. Human Embryo – 6 Weeks of Pregnancy (actual size)

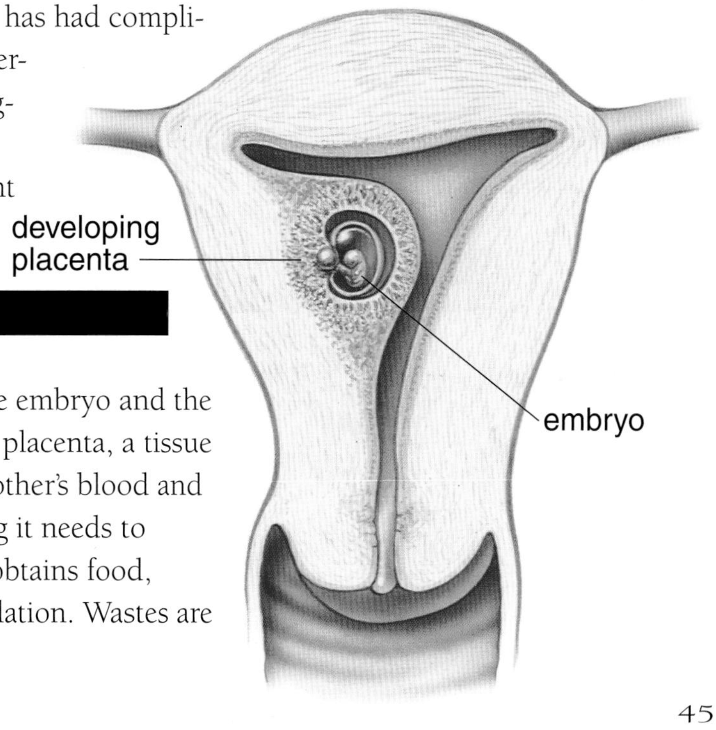

developing placenta

embryo

The Embryo and the Placenta

In the earliest part of the pregnancy, the embryo and the mother's uterus work together creating the placenta, a tissue rich in nutrients that is bathed with the mother's blood and provides the developing embryo everything it needs to thrive. Through the placenta, the embryo obtains food, liquid, and oxygen from the mother's circulation. Wastes are passed through the placenta and discharged by the mother's kidneys. Although the bloodstream of the mother is always separate from the bloodstream of the embryo, the placenta allows them to share intimately their processes of life. Most medicines that the mother takes will enter the embryo through the placental circulation, as will alcohol and drugs. The placenta is an active organ in its own right, secreting human chorionic gonadotropin hormone, estrogen, and progesterone. Among other effects, these hormones signal the ovaries not to release additional eggs during a pregnancy.

The embryo's head and heart are the first to develop, causing the young embryo to look top-heavy. By six weeks of pregnancy, that is, four weeks after ovulation and fertilization, the embryo has a prominent heart, a developing umbilical cord, and buds where the arms and legs will grow. Heart action can be confirmed on an ultrasound after the eighth week of pregnancy.

34. Human Embryo – 10 Weeks of Pregnancy (actual size)

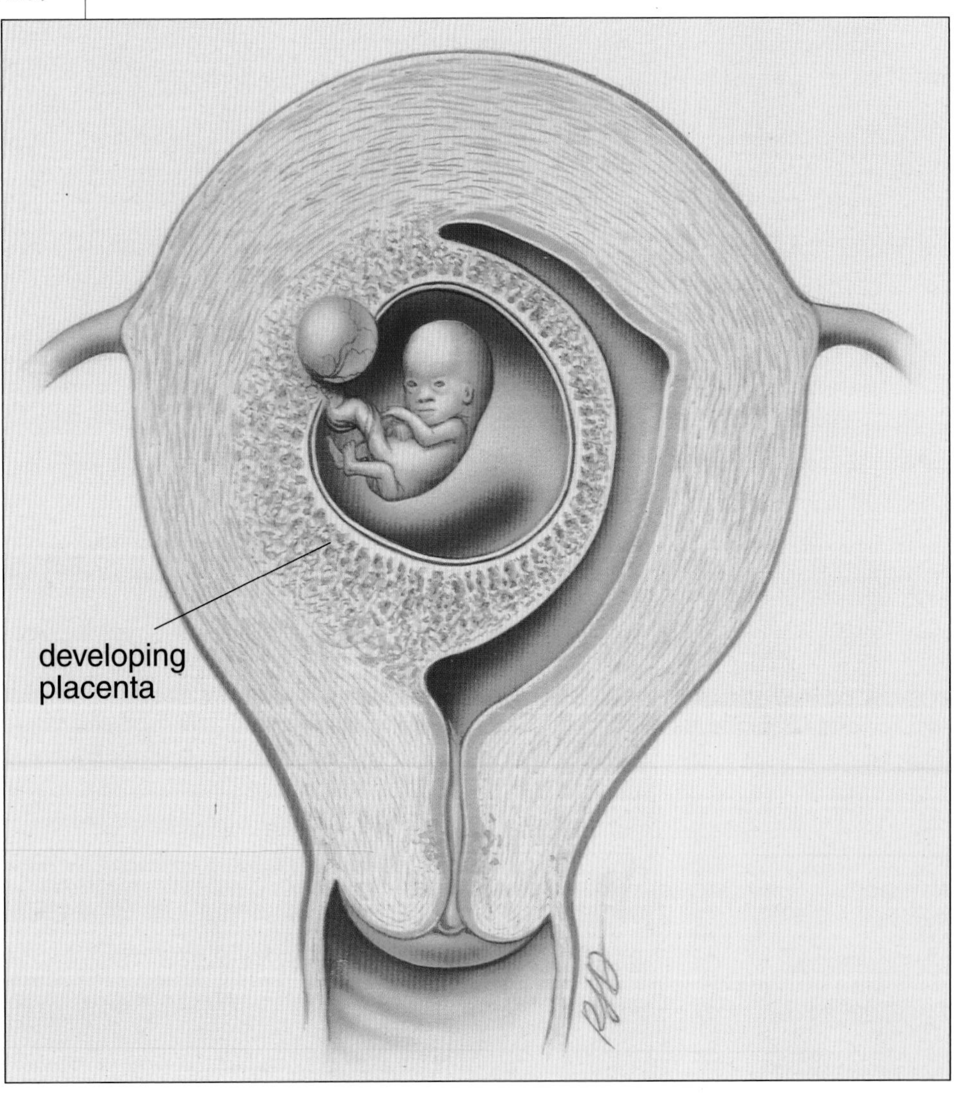

By ten weeks of pregnancy, the embryo has recognizable fingers and toes, ears have appeared, and all major internal organs have begun to develop. It is around one-and-a-half inches in sitting height, the so-called crown-rump length. From this point until birth, the embryo is called the fetus.

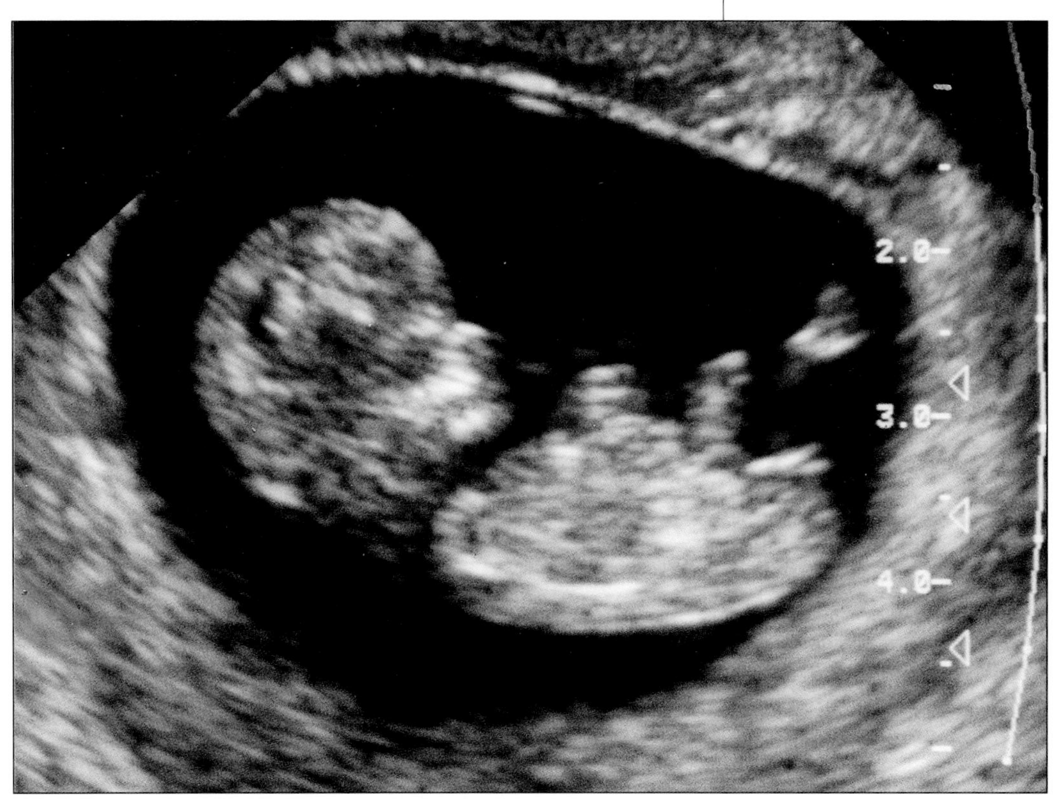

35. Sonogram of 10-11-Week Embryo

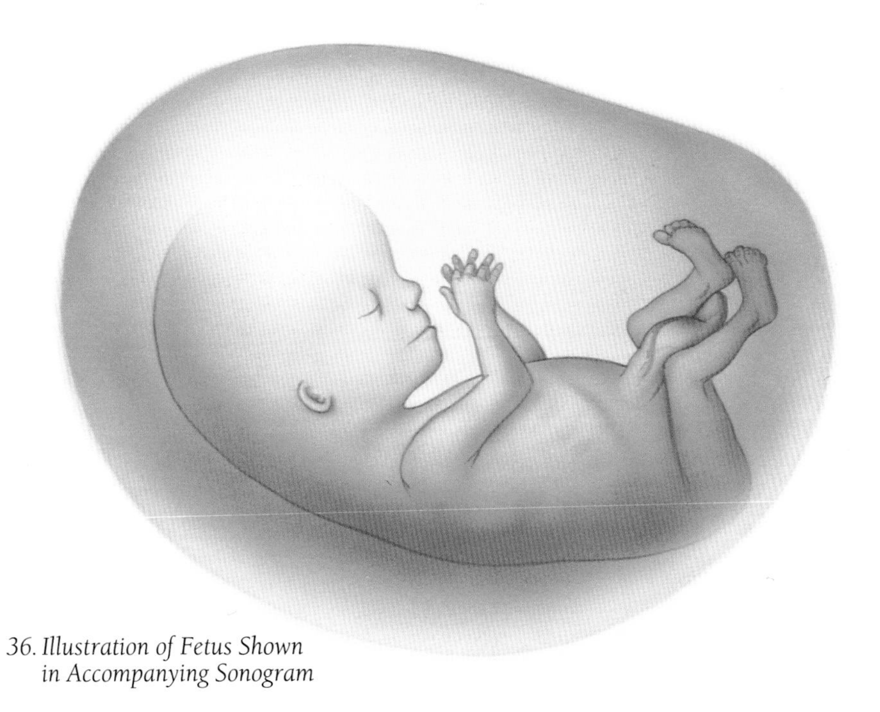

36. Illustration of Fetus Shown in Accompanying Sonogram

Early Fetal Life

The First Trimester

"Miscarriages, also called spontaneous abortions, occur most frequently in the first trimester."

The first trimester of pregnancy extends from fertilization through the twelfth week of pregnancy. During the first trimester, the embryo or fetus begins to develop its organ systems. If the fetus has chromosomal abnormalities, it usually cannot survive beyond the first trimester. Miscarriages, also called spontaneous abortions, occur most frequently in the first trimester. Only 20% of miscarriages occur later in the pregnancy, for example, in cases of some chronic illnesses in the mother. Ten percent of recognized pregnancies miscarry, and it is estimated that around 40% of all pregnancies end in miscarriage, many of them so early that the woman was not even aware that she was pregnant. Additionally, most therapeutic abortions are performed during the first trimester.

The Second Trimester

By the fourteenth week of pregnancy, the uterus can usually be felt upon examination by the doctor or nurse. The fetus is beginning to develop bones and fingernails and toenails, and hair begins to grow. External genitalia can show definite signs of male or female sex. Around four inches long in its sitting height, the fetus is surrounded by amniotic fluid and encased in two membranes, the amniotic membrane and the chorionic sac.

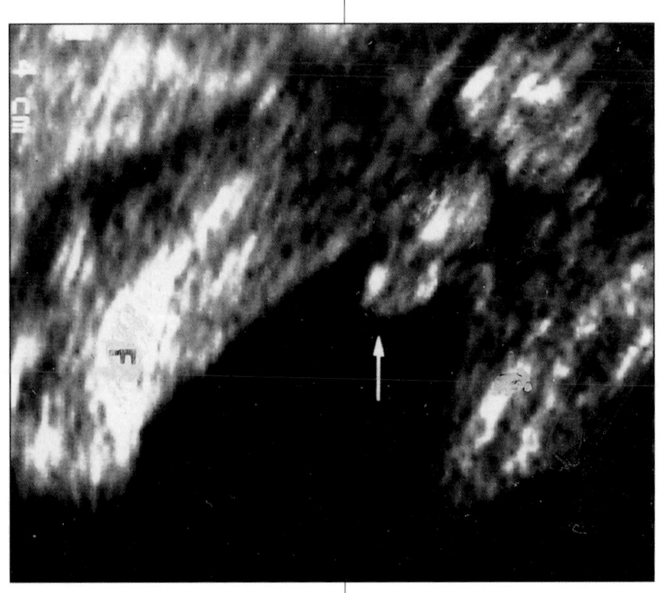

37. Sonogram of 14-Week Fetus Showing Penis

If problems are suspected, amniocentesis can be performed by the fifteenth or sixteenth week. A needle is introduced into the amniotic sac through the mother's abdominal wall. Fluid surrounding the fetus is withdrawn through the needle, and cells that have washed off the fetus are collected for inspection. The chromosomes are then studied to detect hereditary disease or congenital defects in the fetus. In some medical centers, amniocentesis is offered to all women over the age of 35, since the incidence of chromosomal abnor-

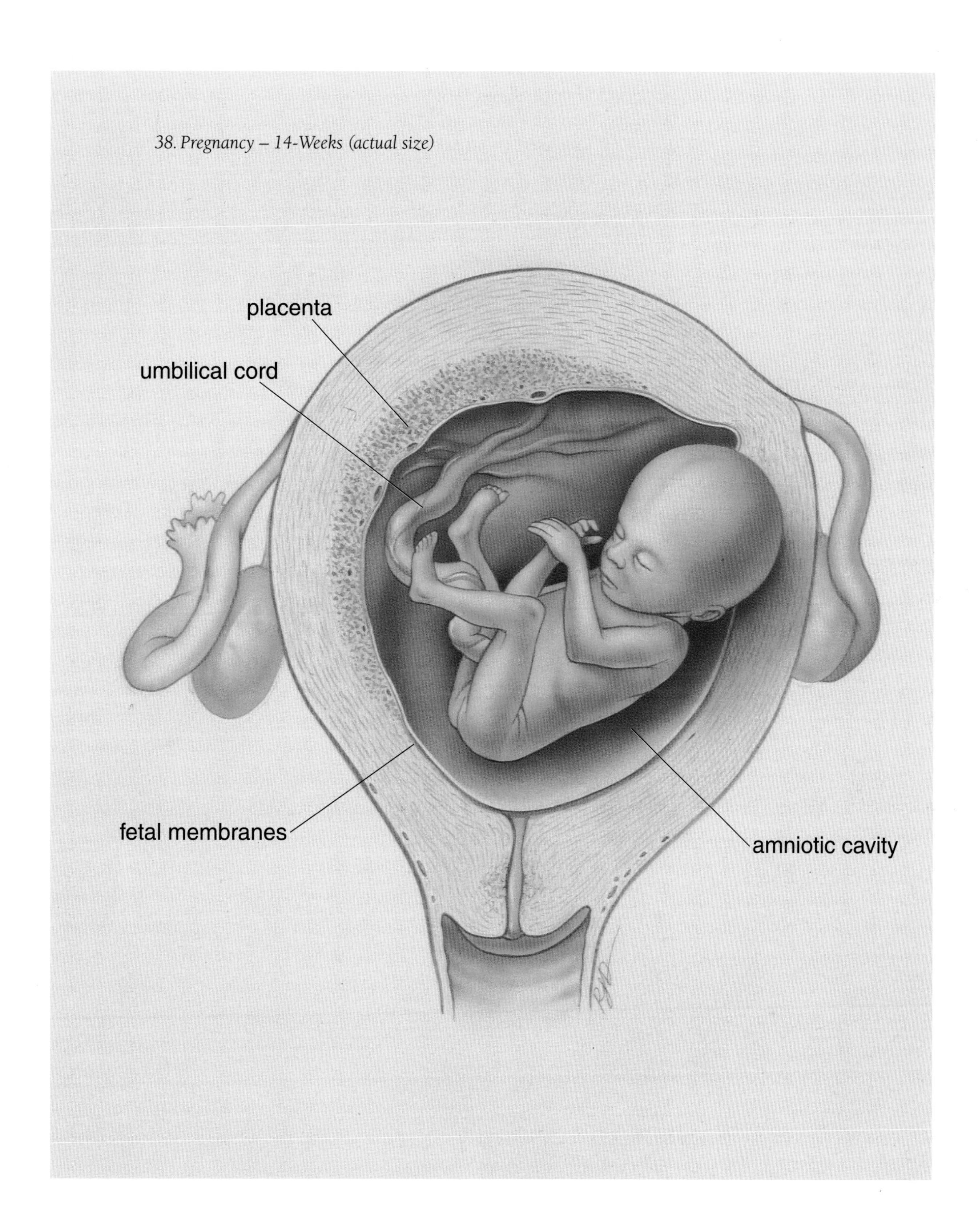
38. Pregnancy – 14-Weeks (actual size)
placenta
umbilical cord
fetal membranes
amniotic cavity

malities in the fetus is higher than the risk of miscarriage following the procedure. As a bonus to the parents, amniocentesis confirms the gender of the fetus.

Through the rest of the second trimester, or mid-trimester, which extends from the 13th week through the 24th week, the fetus continues to mature. Its head and body slowly achieve a more normal-looking proportion. The fetal heartbeat can be heard with a stethoscope applied to the woman's abdomen by the 17th week. By the 20th week, fetal movement is felt.

> ***"The fetal heartbeat can be heard with a stethoscope applied to the woman's abdomen by the 17th week. By the 20th week, fetal movement is felt."***

Recent advances in obstetrics and care of the fetus have provided means to test the blood of the fetus itself. Fetal blood can be sampled by introducing a needle through the mother's abdominal wall, accurately positioning the needle with the help of ultrasound, and actually inserting the needle into the umbilical vein of the fetus. This usually cannot be done before the 23rd week of pregnancy. A fetus with a severe blood disorder can be diagnosed in this manner and can even be given blood transfusions before it is born. Many congenital disorders can be diagnosed in this manner, and some of them are treated surgically while the fetus is still in utero.

At 24 weeks, the crown-rump length is approximately 8 inches and the average fetus weighs 630 grams or close to one-and-a-half pounds. Its eyebrows and eyelids have developed. The skin appears wrinkled because little fat has accumulated under the skin.

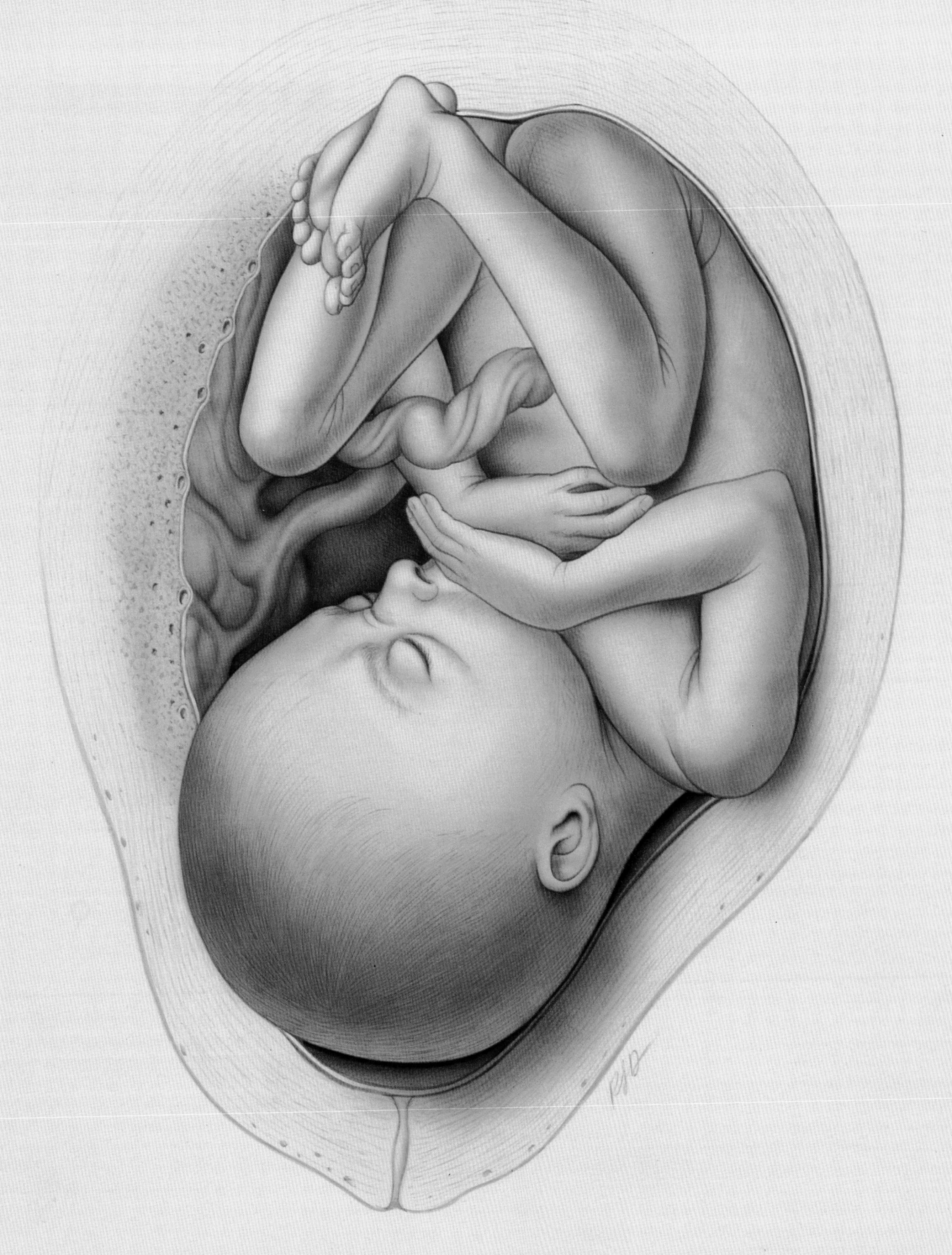

39. 24th Week of Pregnancy (actual size)

Late Fetal Life

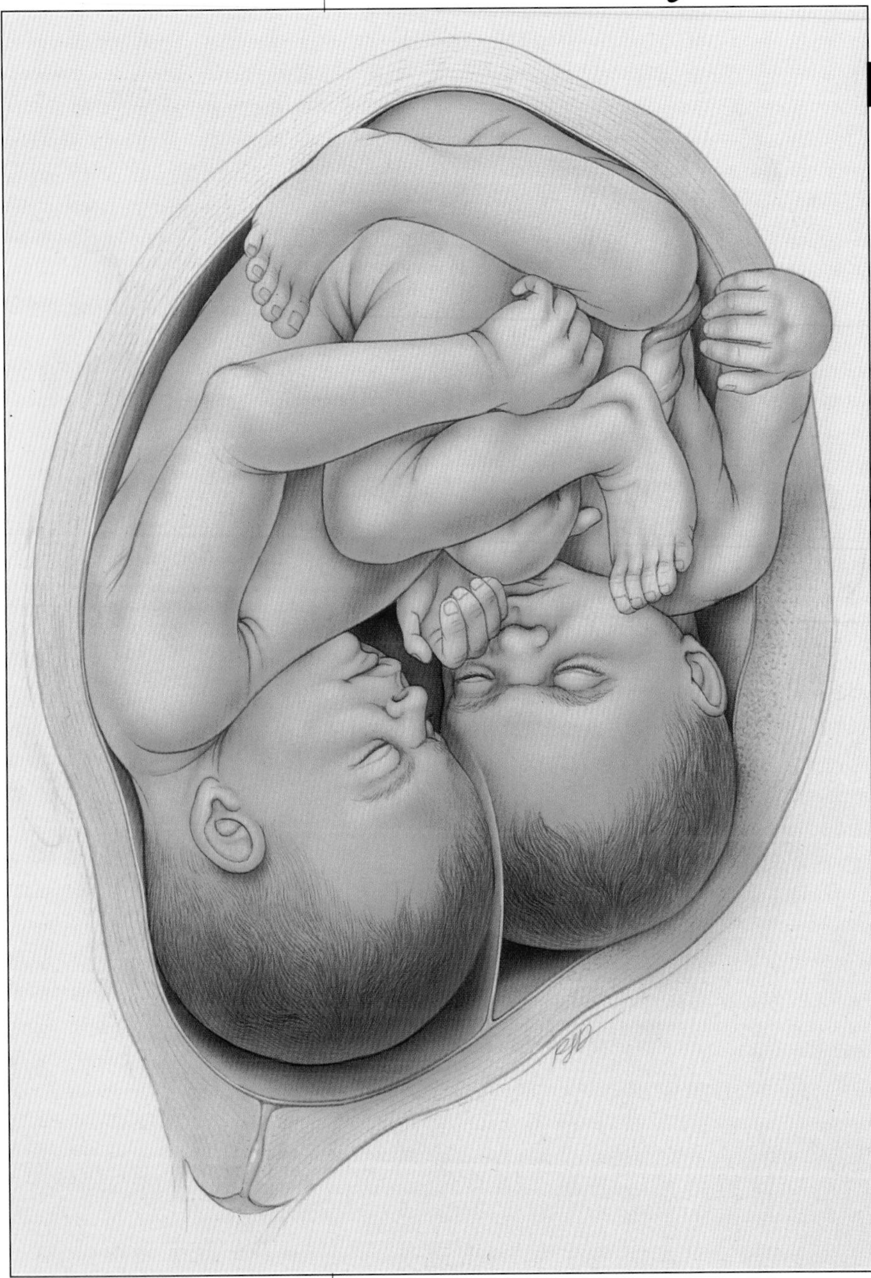

40. Full Term Twins Shown in Uterus

The Third Trimester

The third trimester bridges the stage from fetus to newborn. During these last three months, the fetus grows at an accelerated rate, multiplying its weight by a factor of five and increasing its length by around four-and-a-half inches. A fetus born during the last trimester has a higher survival rate, especially if it receives expert neonatal care. The fetus accumulates what will soon be called "baby fat" during this time, so it appears plump instead of wrinkled. The head remains the largest part of the fetus, and is usually covered with hair. By the 36th or 37th week of pregnancy, the fetal head is usually positioned downward in the mother's uterus, waiting to be born. If twins are developing, they share the mother's uterus, each of them within their own membranous sac.

By the time the fetus has reached term, that is, 40 weeks gestation or 38 weeks from fertilization, it weighs approximately 3,400 grams or nearly seven-and-a-half pounds and is over 14 inches in crown-rump length although some fetuses can be much smaller or much larger than that. The mother's medical condition and nutritional state are the major factors in determining the final weight of the fetus.

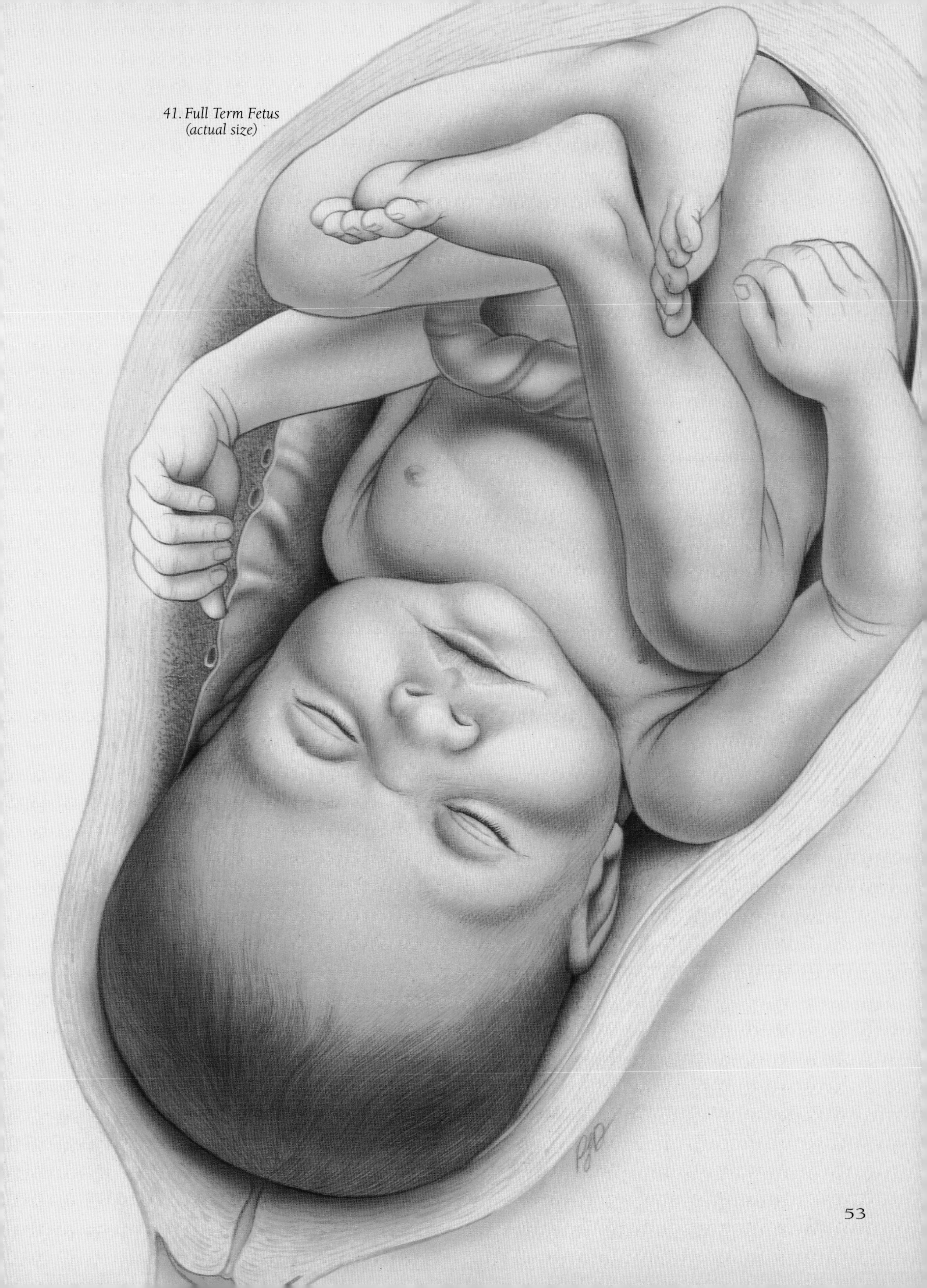

41. *Full Term Fetus*
(actual size)

Maternal Changes in Pregnancy

Throughout the nine months, the mother's body has undergone profound changes. Her life revolves around the developing fetus within her womb.

PHYSICAL CHANGES

The mother's body weight has increased approximately 25 pounds. Her breasts have enlarged dramatically and can be uncomfortably sore at times. Although the nausea experienced by many pregnant women, so-called "morning sickness," usually stops by the fourth month, many other physical changes make the mother feel that her body is no longer her own and, in a manner of speaking, it is not.

"During pregnancy, the mother's blood volume increases by almost 50% with a high percentage of the extra blood circulating directly to the placenta."

As it grows, the uterus takes up almost all the space in the mother's abdomen, pushing aside the intestines and resting against other organs. The weight of the pregnant uterus may cause the mother to experience such symptoms as constipation, heartburn, and backache. Hemorrhoids and varicose veins may develop because the weight of the uterus impedes blood return from the extremities. The mother's metabolism of protein, water, carbohydrates, minerals, and fats changes profoundly. Such changes may result in diabetes that often clears after pregnancy. During pregnancy, the mother's blood volume increases by almost 50% with a high percentage of the extra blood circulating directly to the placenta. There are unexplained changes in the woman's immune system that seem to make her more susceptible to certain infections. The pregnant woman's heart beats faster and stronger. The kidneys grow to accommodate their increased workload. Pregnancy may make the woman appear flushed because blood circulation to the skin increases to discharge the extra heat of her quickened metabolism.

Despite these, at times, uncomfortable changes, the pregnant woman can continue doing pretty much what she wants to do. In times past, pregnant women were confined and restricted, prevented from doing the simplest tasks for fear of injury to her or the fetus. Today, it is known that regular exercise is good for the mother and fetus and that the mother's discomfort is the only factor that should interfere in any activity. Many women continue to work throughout pregnancy. During a normal pregnancy, a healthy woman can continue to travel, to bathe, and to wear whatever clothing feels comfortable.

42. Full Term Fetus in Uterus Showing How it Takes Up Most of the Space in the Mother's Abdomen

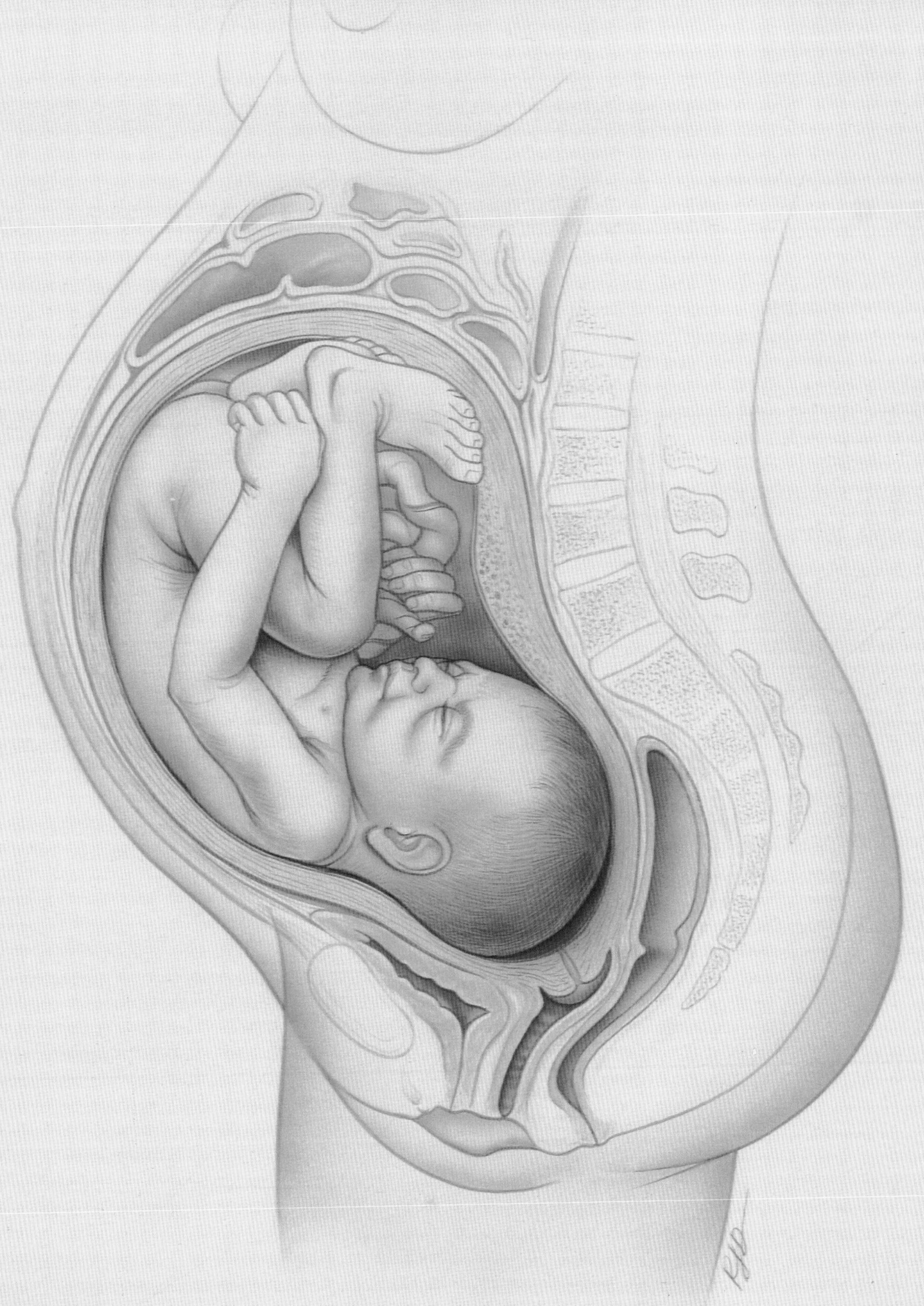

She can have sexual intercourse throughout a normal pregnancy until labor begins or rupture of the membranes occur without fear of harm to the fetus.

LIFE CHANGES

"Despite the physical discomforts of their pregnancy, they are creating a life, extending their family, and taking part in the oldest and most wondrous event of life."

Pregnancy confers some privileges, as well it should. Not only do strangers stop pregnant women to wish them well and offer them seats on public transportation, but such legislated benefits as maternity leave are increasingly common. When the pregnancy is planned and desired, many women feel a heightened sense of happiness and serenity during their pregnancies. When they reflect on the miracle happening within their bodies, they feel awe at their powers. Despite the physical discomforts of their pregnancy, they are creating a life, extending their families, and taking part in the oldest and most wondrous event of life.

The mother and the father will prepare for the arrival of the new baby. Such rituals as choosing the baby's name, preparing older children for their new brother or sister, and furnishing the nursery are enacted by most new parents. The new baby will cause profound changes in the family, and its arrival can help the family to feel its special worth.

Mother, Father, and Child: Labor and Delivery

INITIATION OF LABOR

At 38 to 40 weeks of pregnancy, the uterus begins preparations for birth. Many factors seem to be involved in bringing a pregnancy to an end and initiating the forces of labor and delivery. Hormonal changes in the uterus, increased production of such biological substances as prostaglandins, interleukins, and oxytocin, and such events within the fetus as maturation of the adrenal glands and the brain seem to contribute to the onset of uterine contractions. Since premature delivery is the greatest single factor in infant mortality and complication, control of the onset of labor and delivery is critical to human health. Doctors know that such conditions as infection, fetal abnormalities, an overdistended uterus, fetal death, abnormalities of the cervix or uterus, or serious disease in the mother can result in premature labor. However, there is still great mystery surrounding the question of what triggers normal labor.

Whatever guarantees its proper onset, normal labor and delivery is a biological masterpiece. The baby achieves the head-downward position for birth in most cases, the cervix thins and its opening widens, and the uterus contracts with more and more force. Primiparas, mothers having their first child, ordinarily have longer, more uncomfortable labors than multiparas, women who have already given birth. Once a woman has had children, her uterus and cervix have become seasoned to labor and delivery, and the events usually take less time.

THE FATHER'S ROLE

The father plays a central role in preparation for labor and in the delivery room. The father's life, too, has been profoundly changed during his partner's pregnancy. Although his body does not reflect the coming changes in his life, his relationship with his wife or lover has been altered dramatically to make room for the awaited child. The more the father can learn about pregnancy and labor, the more helpful he will be as a coach. Hospitals routinely allow fathers to be present at the birth of their children. They help the delivery to be smoother and they, too, can bond with their child from the very first moment of its life.

"The more the father can learn about pregnancy and labor, the more helpful he will be as a coach."

First Stage of Labor

Labor is conventionally divided into three stages. The first stage begins with the onset of regular uterine contractions and lasts until the cervix is fully dilated, that is, until the opening to the womb has stretched to its fullest, usually around 10 centimeters or 4 inches in diameter. Dilatation, or stretching, of the lower birth canal is usually associated with deep pelvic pain and backache. This stage usually lasts around twelve to sixteen hours for primiparas or six to eight hours for multiparas. In special circumstances, such as a large fetus or particularly weak uterine contractions, it can take significantly longer than that.

"The opening of the cervix and its thickness will be measured regulary to make sure that labor is proceeding normally. If the labor slows down during this stage, the hormone oxytocin may be administered to strengthen the uterine contractions."

During the first stage of labor, the mother will be examined and the position of the fetus will be checked. The obstetrician or midwife will determine the level of engagement of the fetus, that is, the degree to which it has dropped into the mother's pelvic canal. The opening of the cervix and its thickness will be measured regularly to make sure that labor is proceeding normally. If the labor slows down during this stage, the hormone oxytocin may be administered to strengthen the uterine contractions. The mother will be asked not to eat solid foods during her labor to prevent complications of vomiting should she need general anesthesia. She will be allowed to walk around until the membranes rupture, that is, until her waters break. If she is experiencing undue pain, she is offered a form of pain relief once her contractions have been established and the cervix has begun to dilate.

The fetal heartbeat will be monitored regularly throughout labor. If the fetal heartbeat slows down after a uterine contraction, the fetus may be in distress and may need help. In high-risk situations, like a premature birth or a chronically ill mother, the fetus will be monitored electronically, either with electrodes outside the mother's abdomen or with sensors placed on the fetal head, to obtain minute-to-minute recordings of the fetal heartbeat and the strength of the uterine contractions.

43. First Stage of Labor

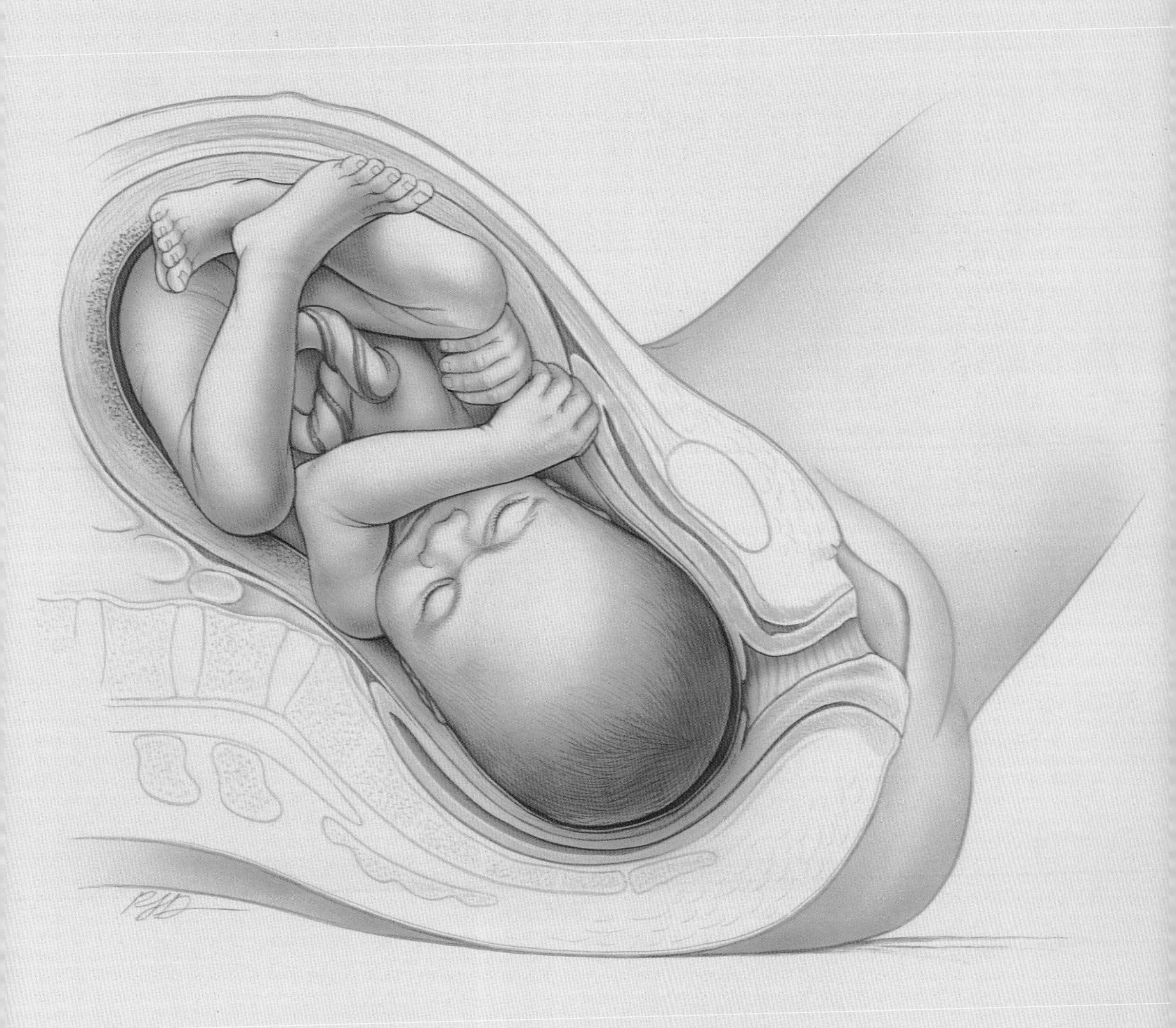

Second Stage of Labor

Preparation for the Birth

"This is the part of labor in which the mother has to work very hard, pushing with her abdominal muscles to help the baby move through the birth canal."

The second stage of labor, usually the shortest, extends from full dilatation of the cervix to the actual birth of the baby. The second stage usually takes around a half-hour, although for first pregnancies, it may take up to two hours. The contractions come about every minute, and also last around a minute. This is the part of labor in which the mother has to work very hard, pushing with her abdominal muscles to help the baby move through the birth canal.

At this stage, the fetal heartbeat is checked by the doctor or midwife very frequently, especially if there are any risks. If the fetus appears distressed or if the uterine contractions slow down ominously, the baby can be delivered with the use of obstetrical forceps or by Cesarean section.

As the baby descends into the birth canal, its head is usually bent toward its chest. In a breech presentation, that is, a feet-first delivery, the hips may be the first to be seen. The doctor or midwife will insure that the baby does not come out too quickly. He or she will place a hand on the part of the baby coming out first to prevent tearing of the mother's tissue by the baby. In most cases, a small surgical cut called an episiotomy is made in the mother's vulva if it appears that the delivery will make a tear in her tissues.

The birthing mother is helped into a position to make it easiest for the baby to complete its journey. She may remain on her back with her legs bent slightly and somewhat elevated or she may rest on her side. Some women find it most comfortable to assume a squatting position for the actual birth, and midwives in many parts of the world deliver babies with the mothers in this position.

The Birth Itself

In a head-first birth, called a vertex presentation, the baby's scalp will be seen at the cervix. When the top of the baby's head is seen in the cervical opening, it is said to have crowned. As the head maneuvers into the birth canal, it usually rotates into a face-down position, fitting the slimmest dimension of the head to the narrowest dimension of the pelvic bones. As the head begins to emerge, it usually starts to extend, that is, to pick up its chin. At this point, the doctor or nurse

44. Beginning of Second Stage of Labor

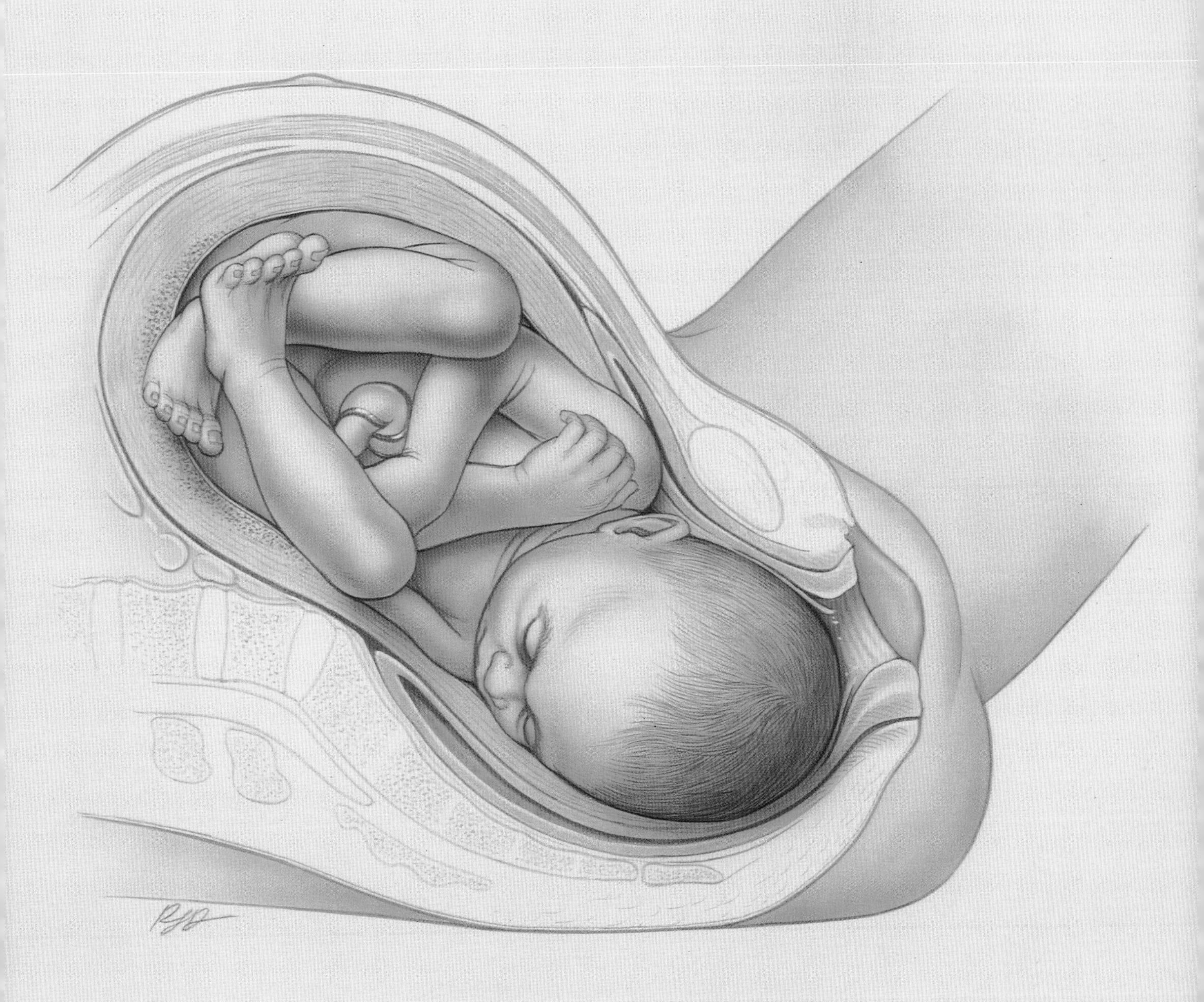

45. *Second Stage of Labor Continuing*

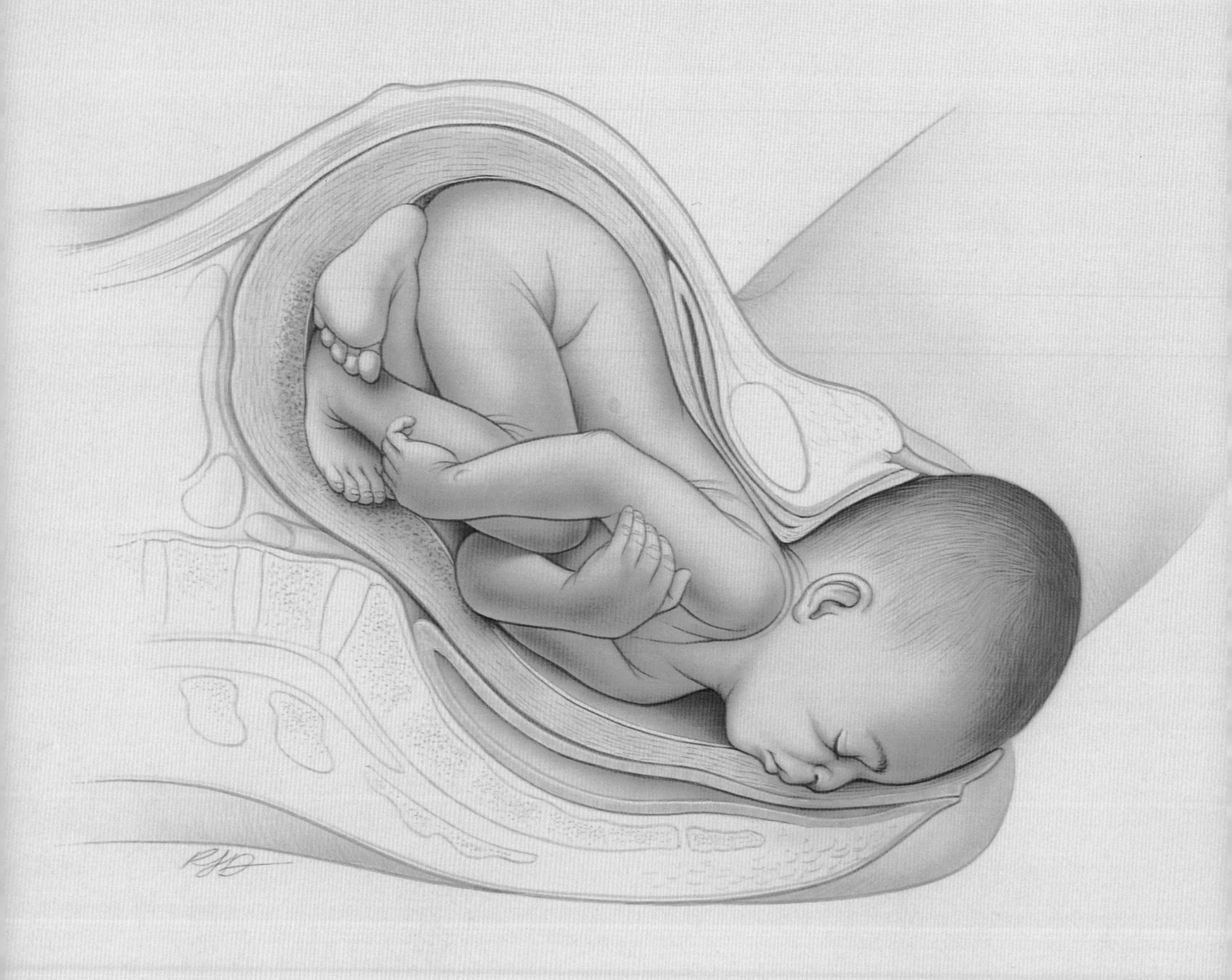

46. Delivery of Head and Shoulders

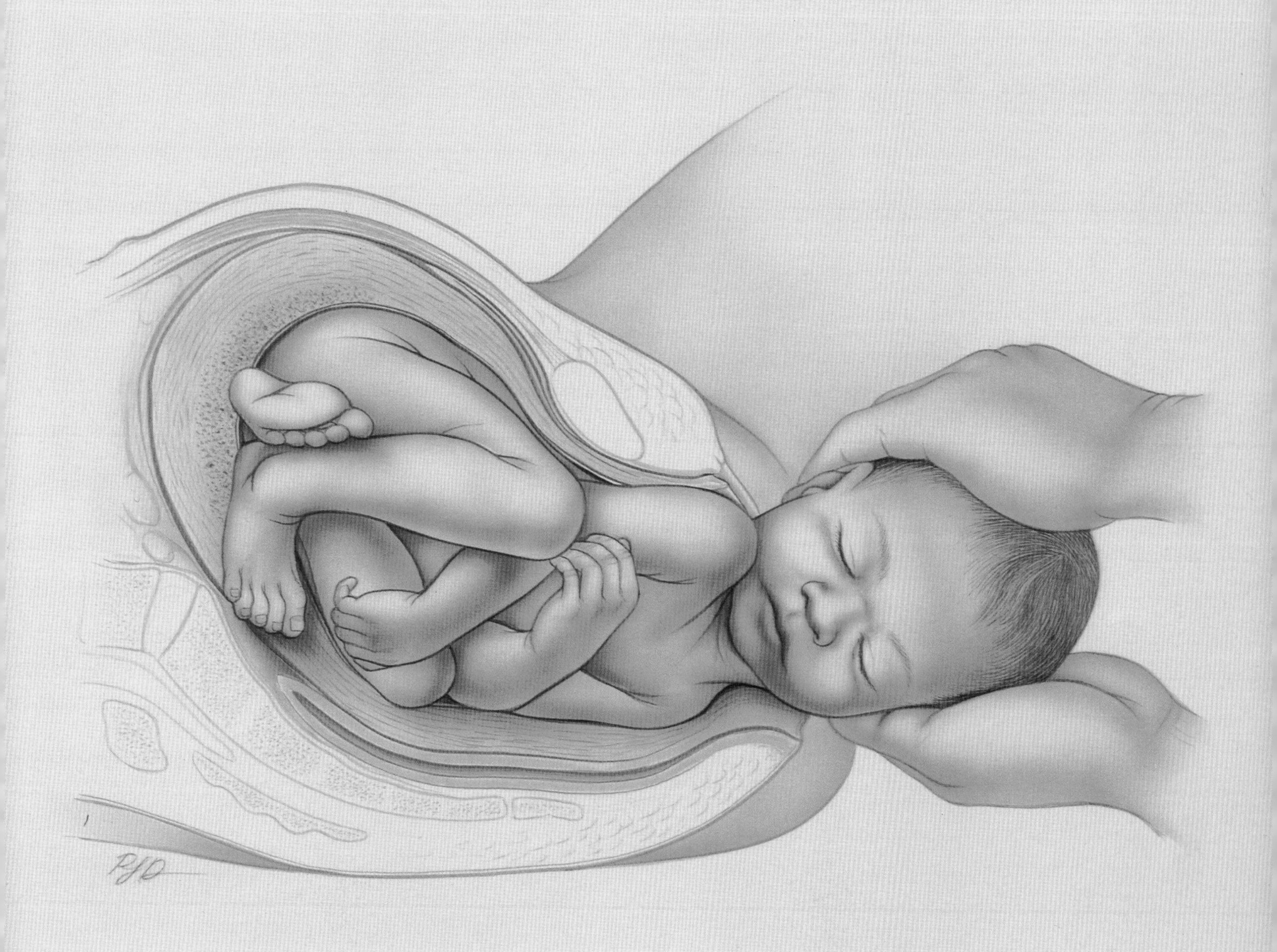

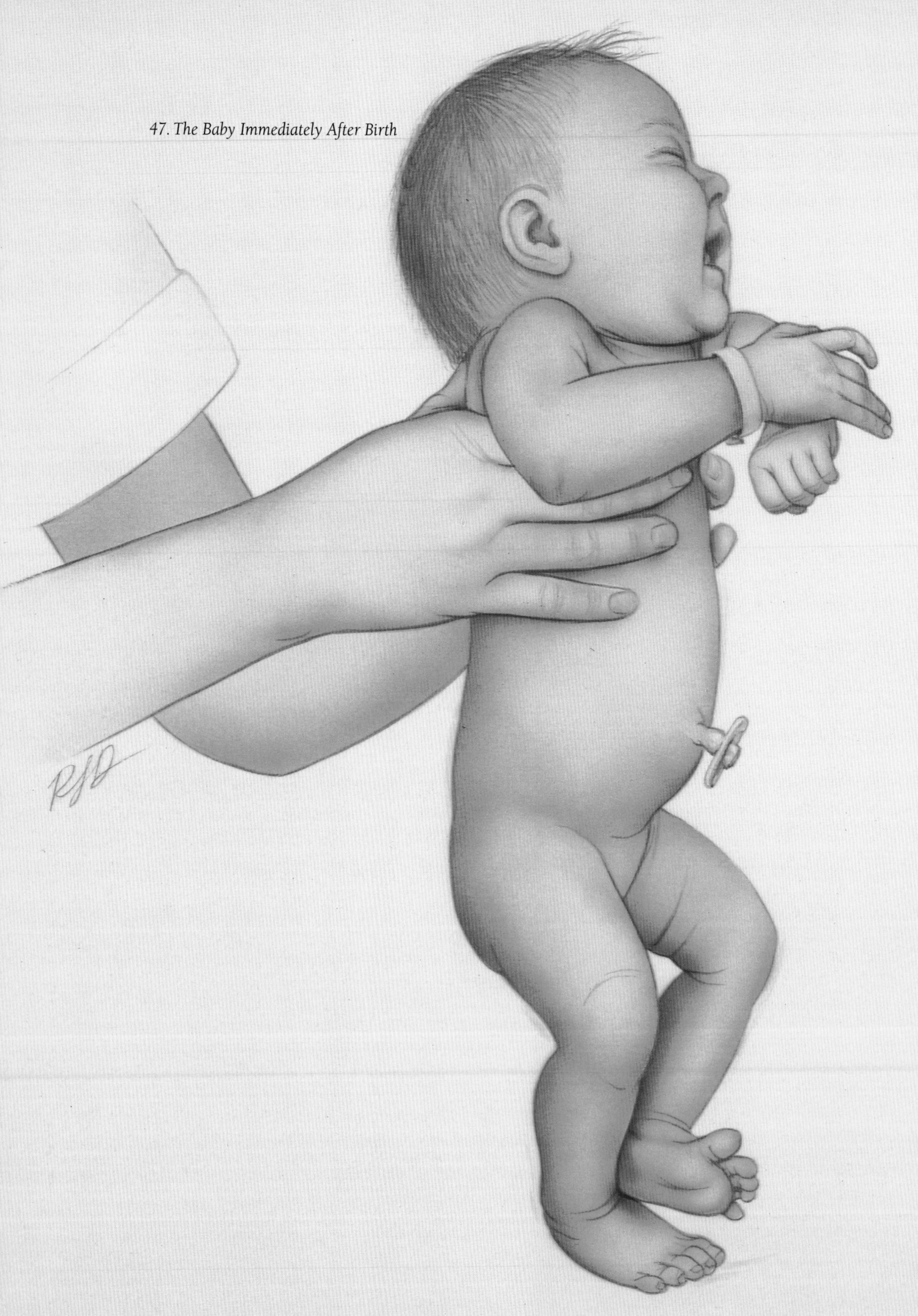

47. The Baby Immediately After Birth

may have to help tilt the head toward the back to allow the baby's head to clear the mother's pelvic bones.

No matter how many deliveries one has seen, the emergence of the baby's head from the vagina is an amazing and moving sight. The brand-new infant is fully in the world for the first time, and what a privilege it is to help bring him or her into the world safely. The mother and father will feel tremendously strong emotions as the child moves out of the vagina into the waiting world and they see their own child in the light of day.

Things happen quickly, though, and the doctor or nurse does not have much time for reflection. The head will ordinarily rotate back to its original position facing one side as soon as it clears the vulva. The baby's neck will be checked to make sure the umbilical cord is not wrapped around it, and if it is there, it is moved. The nose and mouth are gently cleansed of any fluid that may make it difficult for the baby to breathe.

Ordinarily, the shoulders follow delivery of the head spontaneously. Sometimes, the doctor or midwife needs to exert slight downward pressure to help the shoulders clear the vaginal opening. The baby is then held by the person attending the delivery as the mother makes one last push to bring out the hips and legs of the baby. The baby is gently wiped dry and examined to make sure breathing starts. Babies are not routinely held by their heels and spanked anymore. The umbilical cord is clamped and cut once its blood has drained into the baby. The baby is then given to the mother and father to hold.

"As the head maneuvers into the birth canal, it usually rotates into a face-down position, fitting the slimmest dimension of the head to the narrowest dimension of the pelvic bones."

48. Third Stage of Labor

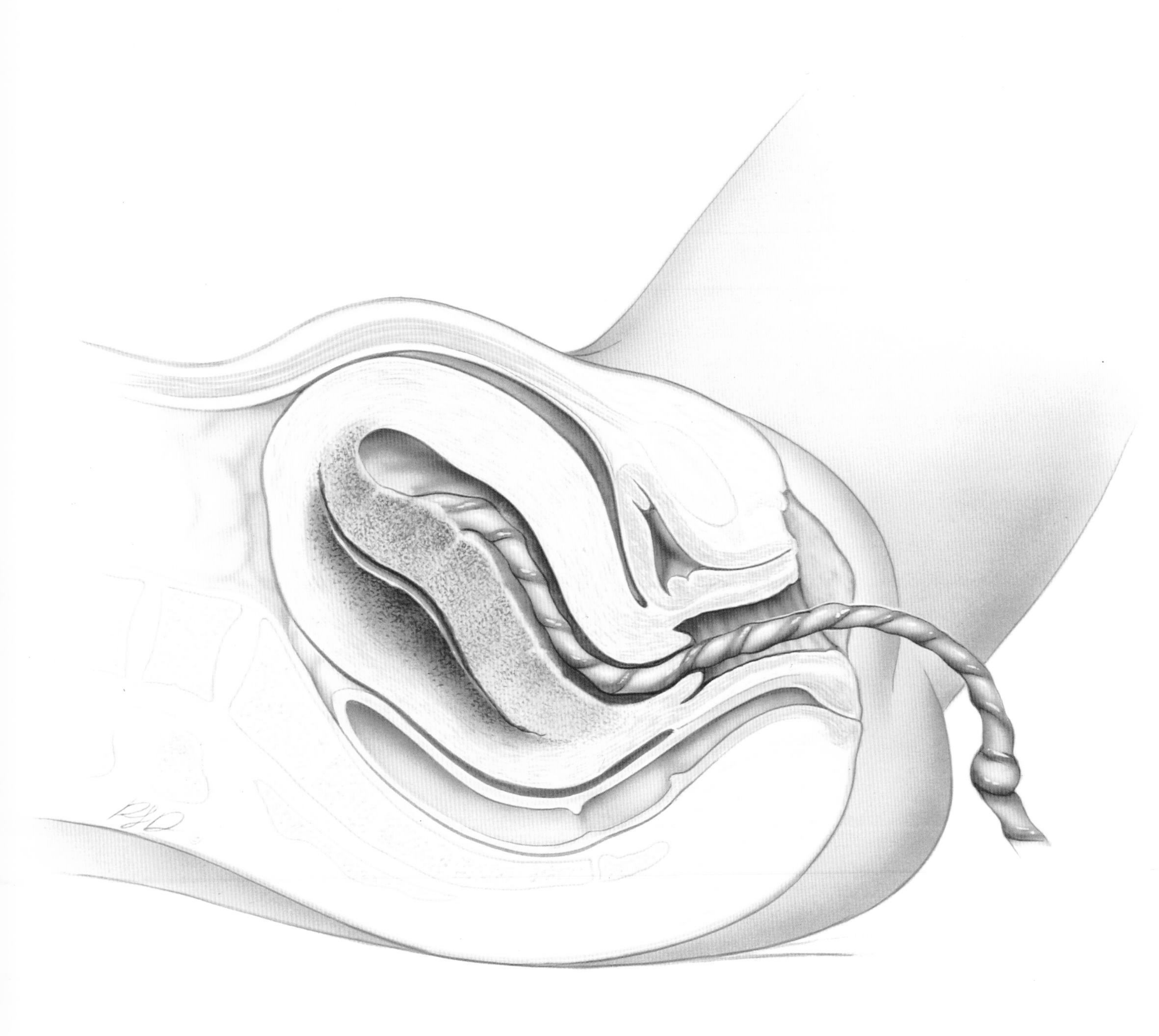

Third Stage of Labor

The third and final stage of labor is the delivery of the placenta and fetal membranes, also called the afterbirth. In general, the afterbirth is delivered without assistance within ten to fifteen minutes following the birth of the baby.

Sometimes, gentle pressure is needed to completely remove the membranes. The uterus continues to contract to expel the placenta, and a hand held lightly on the uterus can confirm this. Pressure should not be applied on the uterus to make the placenta expel. Ordinarily there is some vaginal bleeding as the placenta separates from the inside of the uterus. If the placenta does not deliver spontaneously, the doctor or midwife may need to examine the inside of the uterus to help remove it. During the third stage of labor, the mother will be examined for cervical or vaginal lacerations. Oxytocin or other hormones may be administered following the delivery of the placenta to help control the normal uterine bleeding. If an episiotomy has been performed, it will be repaired at the end of the third stage.

"In general, the afterbirth is delivered without assistance within ten to fifteen minutes following the birth of the baby."

49. Lactating Breast, Sectioned to Show Glands

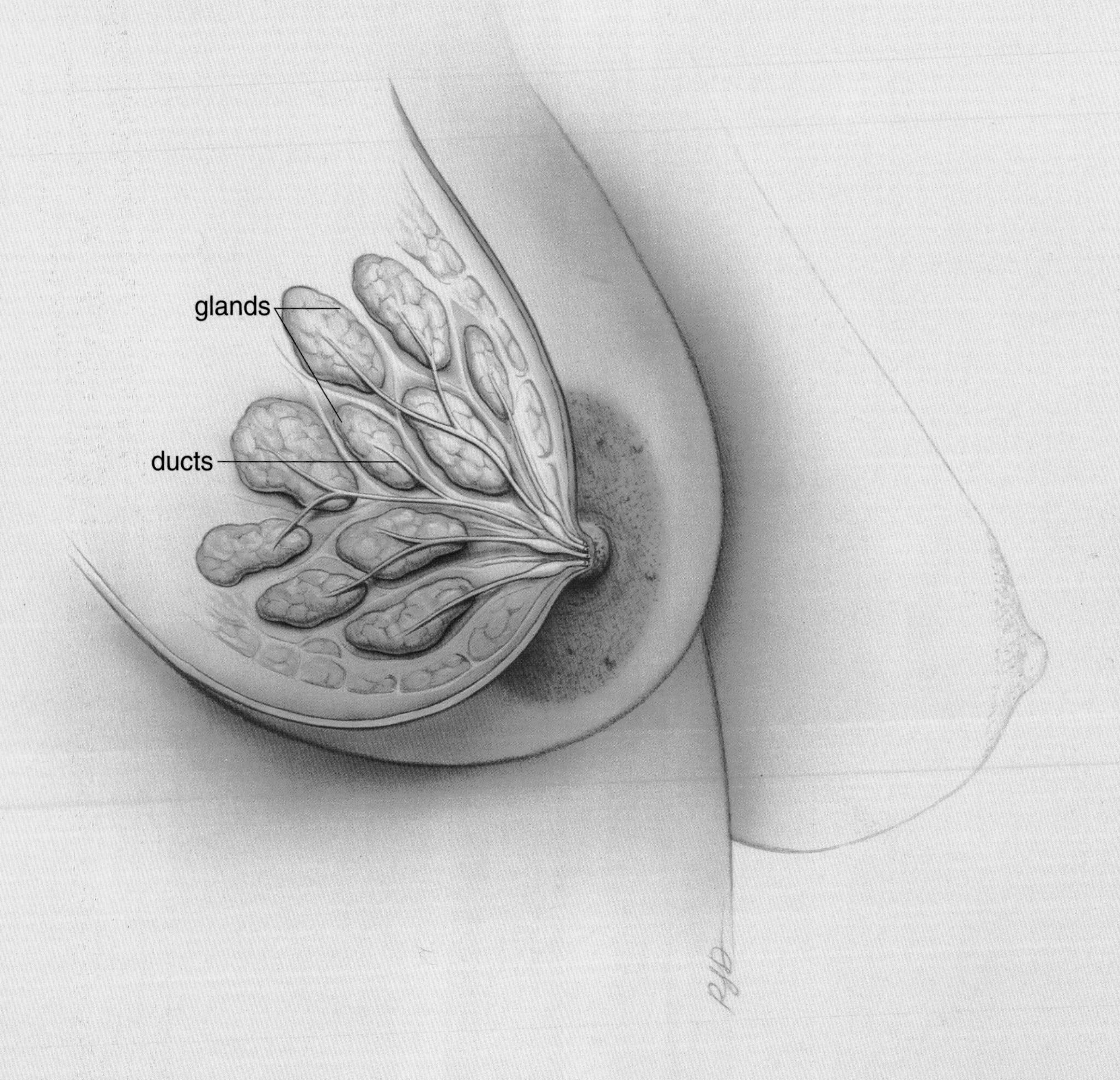

Lactation and Breast-Feeding

MILK PRODUCTION

Throughout pregnancy, the breast tissue has been preparing to feed the infant. As the breasts swell, they also become enriched in milk glands. The hormones of pregnancy, estrogen and progesterone, encourage the development of milk glands and ducts. Women's breasts may secrete a thin fluid called colostrum even before the delivery of the child.

When the levels of estrogen and progesterone fall dramatically after the birth, the effects of another hormone called prolactin determine breast function. Prolactin directly stimulates milk production in the breast tissue. When the infant is allowed to suckle at the nipples, oxytocin is released from the mother's pituitary gland. This hormone enables the milk to be delivered to the nipples where the infant can drink. Mothers can begin breast-feeding within the first few hours of birth. Lactation also suppresses ovulation in most cases and therefore may prevent another pregnancy from beginning, leading to a natural form of spacing of children.

"When the levels of estrogen and progesterone fall dramatically after the birth, the effects of another hormone called prolactin determine breast function."

ADVANTAGES OF BREAST-FEEDING

The advantages of breast-feeding for mother and infant are well-known. Breast milk is an ideal biological food for the infant, containing almost all the minerals and vitamins the baby needs. In addition, the mother's immunity to infections may pass via the milk into the infant, protecting him or her from infectious illnesses. Perhaps most importantly, breast-feeding begins the mother and child on an intimate physical relationship that deepens their attachment.

Some reasons a mother would not want to breast-feed are the presence of such illnesses as hepatitis, HIV infection, or breast cancer. Some types of breast surgery prevent milk production or delivery, therefore making breast-feeding impossible. If the mother has to take medications that would get into the breast milk and harm the baby, she should not breast-feed. Finally, some women are unable to fit regular breast-feeding into a schedule.

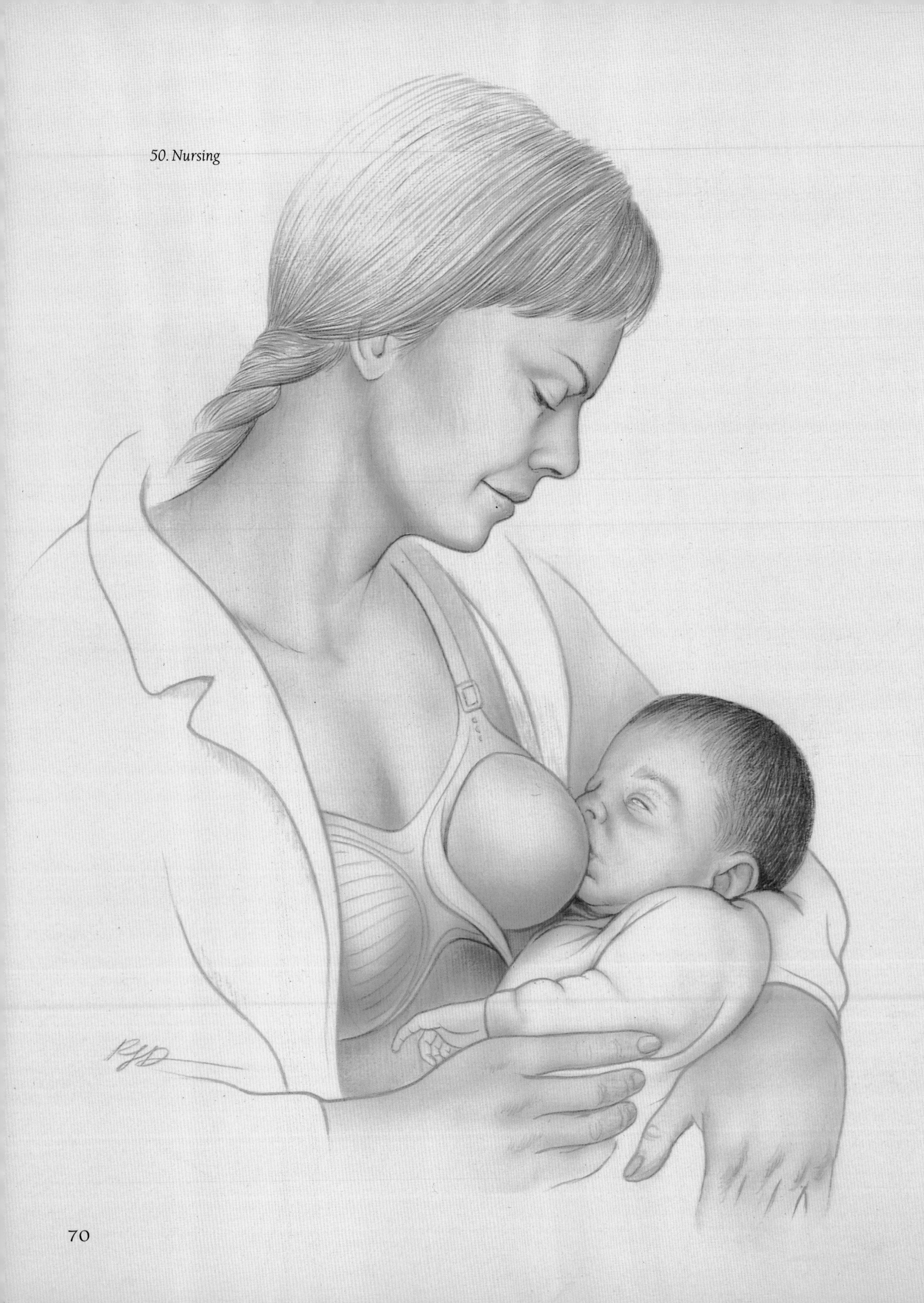

50. Nursing

Man and Woman: Contraception

One of the most important features of a successful pregnancy is that it is planned and wanted. A couple may choose to use a form of birth control to wait until they are ready for children before getting pregnant. Many methods exist to allow men, women, or couples to control their fertility. Pregnancy can be prevented by inhibiting ovulation, by blocking the sperm from traveling to the egg, or by interfering with implantation. No method except abstinence, that is, not having sex, is 100% effective. If used conscientiously, the methods described here can prevent all but a small number of pregnancies. The choice of birth control method depends on the state of health of the woman, the ability to pay for care, the pregnancy-free time desired, the couple's religious beliefs, and the man's and woman's lifestyle and preferences. Individuals or couples should make decisions about birth control methods in consultation with their gynecologist or urologist, as most of the available methods require a doctor's examination, prescription, and judgment. Effectiveness of any method varies from individual to individual.

"Natural" Methods

The so-called rhythm method relies on the calendar of the menstrual cycle to limit intercourse to nonfertile days of the month. Since fertilization can only occur within two to three days of ovulation, a couple may choose to have sex only on the days when the woman is not fertile. Theoretically, pregnancy should not occur if intercourse is avoided from days 9 to 17, counting from the first day of the menstrual period. However, many women's periods are irregular and the actual timing of ovulation is never totally predictable.

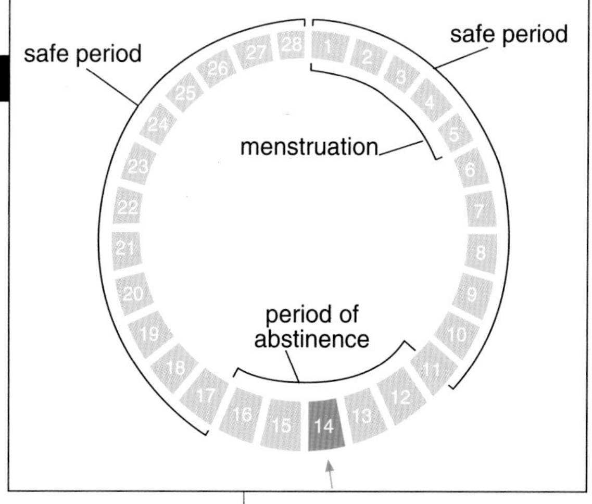

51. Rhythm System for a 28-day Cycle

A rough guide to the time of ovulation is available by counting ahead from a period. Ovulation should occur 14 days after the first day of a period. In addition to counting the days since the last period, a woman can check at least two other physical characteristics to find out when she ovulates. The cervical mucus appears different on the days immediately surrounding ovulation. Ordinarily scanty, thick, and opaque, the mucus becomes abundant, clear, and silky at the time of ovulation.

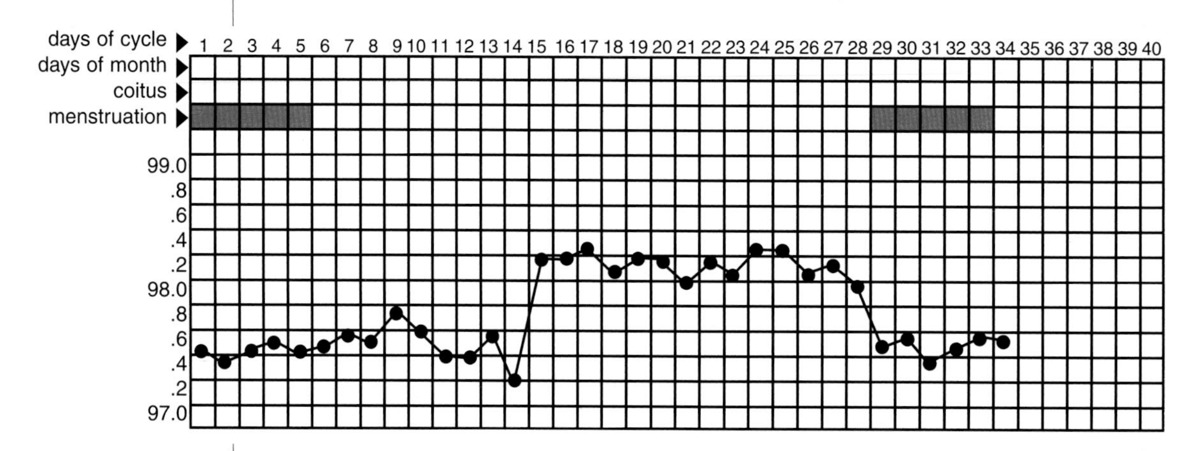

52. Basal Body Temperature Graph

The woman can also check her body temperature every day. If she checks her temperature accurately first thing in the morning with a special thermometer called a basal body thermometer, a woman can detect a slight rise in body temperature of around 0.5 to 0.7 degrees Fahrenheit that signifies that ovulation has taken place. Despite these precautions, irregular cycles make this method of birth control relatively ineffective and unpredictable.

BARRIER METHODS

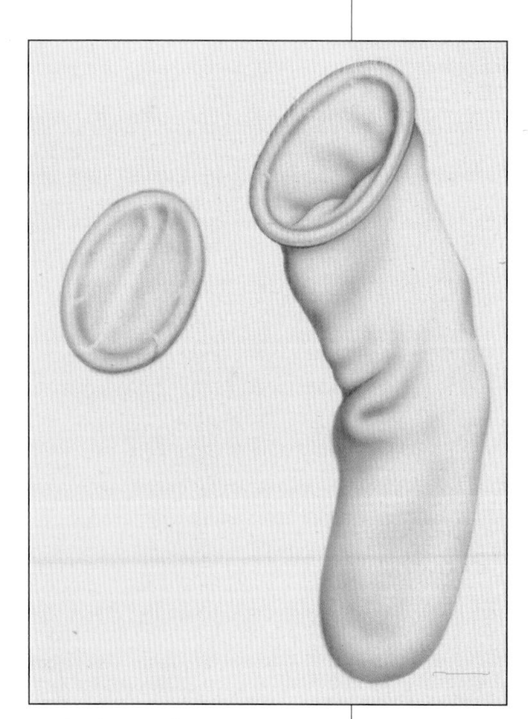

53. The Condom

A number of birth-control methods place a mechanical barrier between the sperm and egg to prevent fertilization. These methods include the male condom, the female condom, the diaphragm, the cervical sponge, and the cervical cap. The barrier methods are generally used along with a spermicide, a cream or foam containing a chemical, that kills any sperm that may get through the barrier.

The male condom is a latex, rubber, or plastic sheath that fits over the distended penis. Condoms are available in many textures and generally are treated with a spermicide chemical. In addition to acting as a barrier against sperm, the condom can prevent the passage of infectious agents from a man to his partner. The increasing prevalence of the human immunodeficiency virus (HIV) that causes AIDS makes the use of the condom critical for all but completely monogamous, healthy partners. The condom can also prevent the spread of hepatitis, syphilis, and gonorrhea.

The disadvantages to the use of the condom for birth control are that it may interfere in the pleasure of sexual intercourse, it sometimes breaks during intercourse, the man must be relied on to place it correctly over the penis before penetration, and it must be carefully removed after intercourse so that semen does not escape into the vagina. When used properly, the condom can be quite effective in preventing pregnancy, but many couples have trouble following all the rules of condom use.

The female condom has been recently introduced into practice. Many women want the protection afforded by the condom but do not trust their male partners to use the male condom effectively. The female condom is a plastic or latex covering that the woman inserts into the vagina prior to intercourse. It has not been in use long enough for its effectiveness to be well studied.

The cervical diaphragm is a barrier method used by the woman to prevent the sperm from entering the cervix. A gynecologist has to fit the woman with her diaphragm, as the sizes of the vagina and the cervix vary widely and the diaphragm must fit snugly to be effective. The diaphragm is a rubber dome whose springy edges will snap into place in the vagina at the level of the cervix, resting between the symphysis pubis in front and the posterior fornix of the vagina in the back.

Smeared with spermicidal cream or gel before placement, the diaphragm must be inserted no more than six hours before intercourse and must remain in place for six hours after intercourse.

If repeated intercourse takes place, the spermicidal preparation must be reapplied with a vaginal applicator.

Neither the woman nor her partner ordinarily feels the diaphragm when it is positioned properly. The diaphragm can also be used to catch menstrual flow if the couple wishes to have intercourse during the woman's period. The diaphragm can be quite effective in preventing pregnancy, depending on the skill with which the woman uses it.

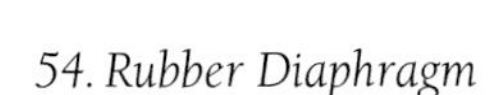

54. Rubber Diaphragm

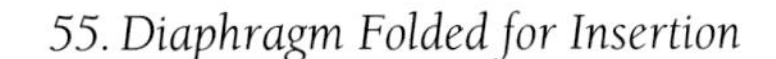

55. Diaphragm Folded for Insertion

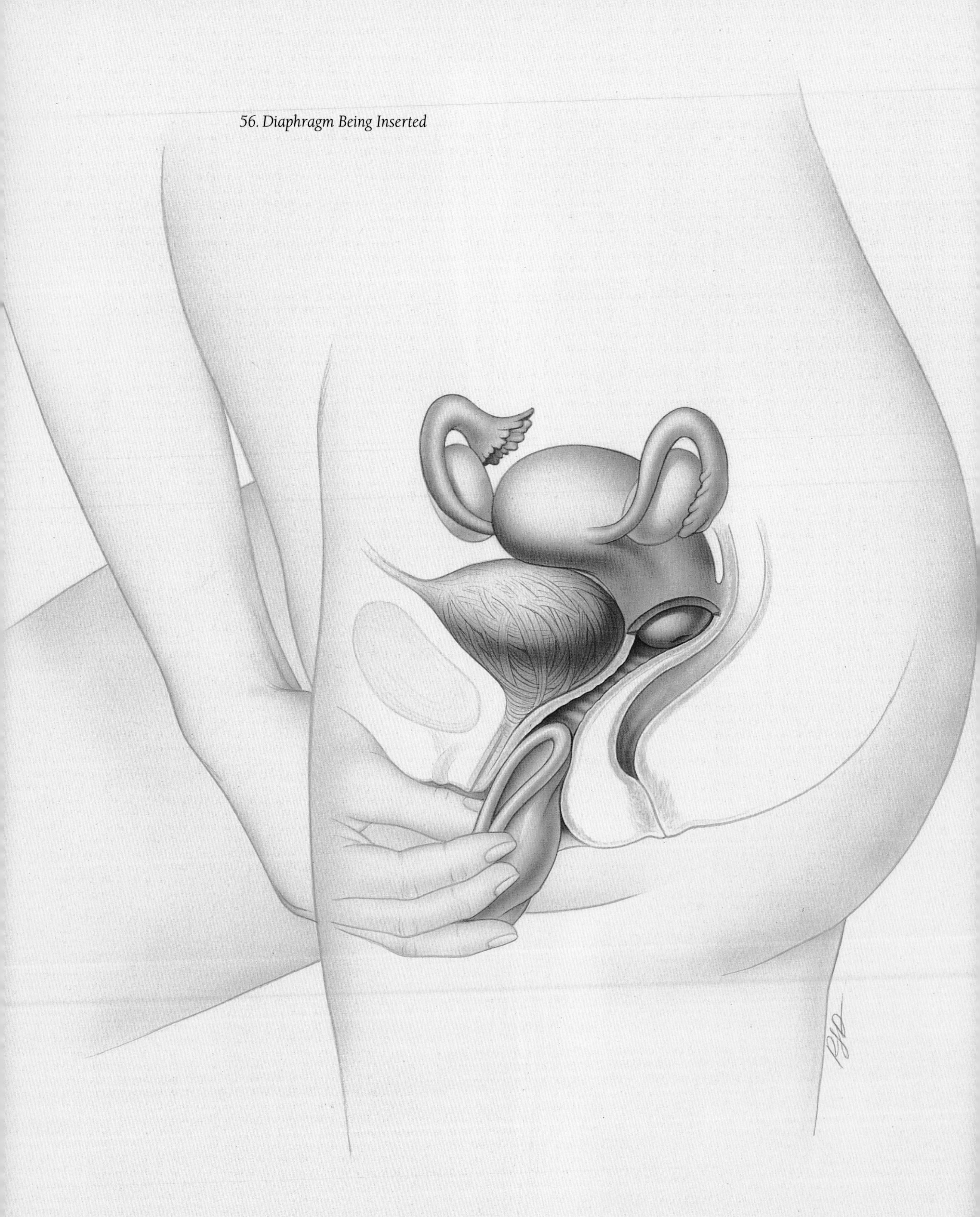

56. Diaphragm Being Inserted

57. Diaphragm in Position

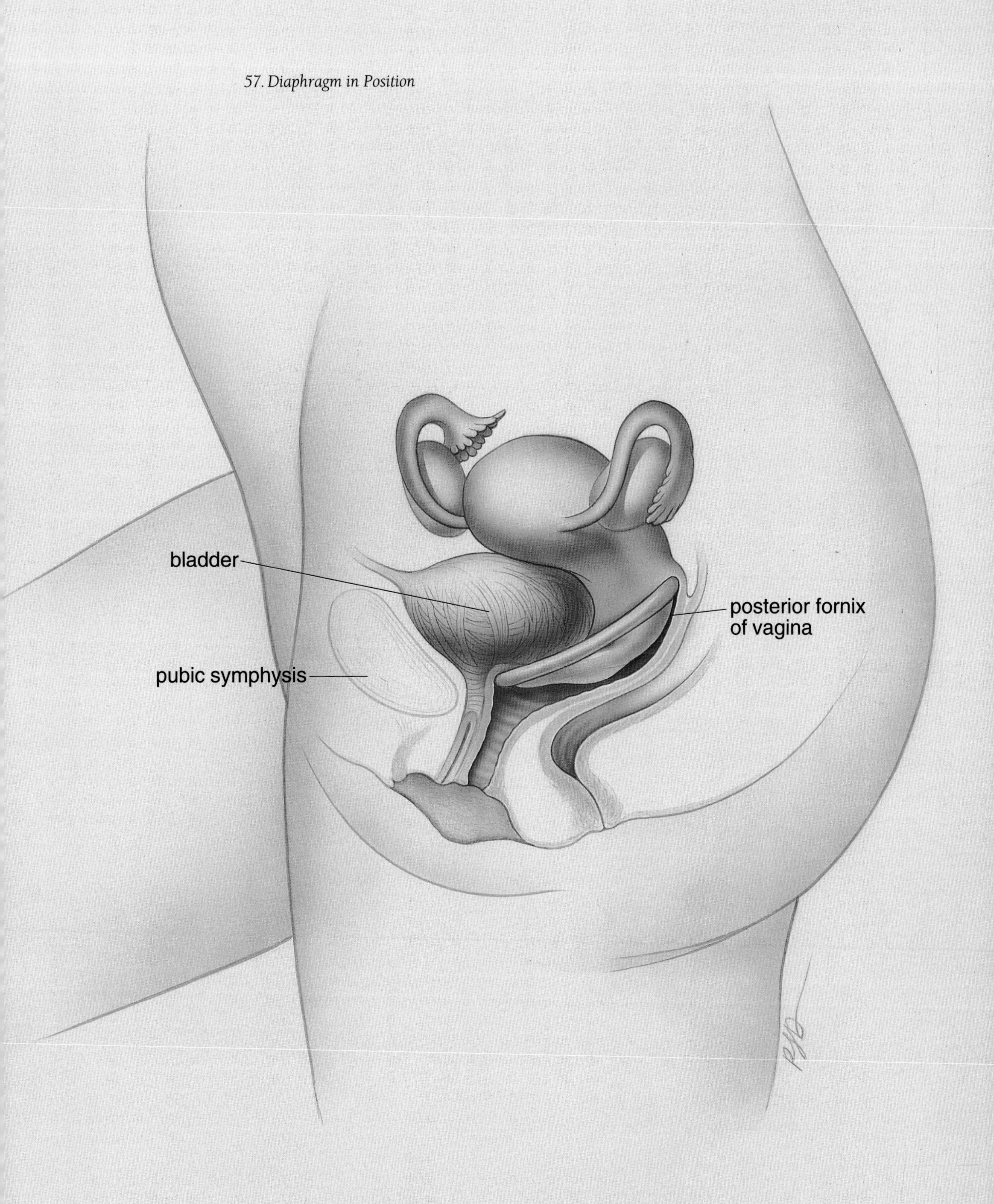

58. Applying a Spermicidal Preparation After Diaphragm is in Place

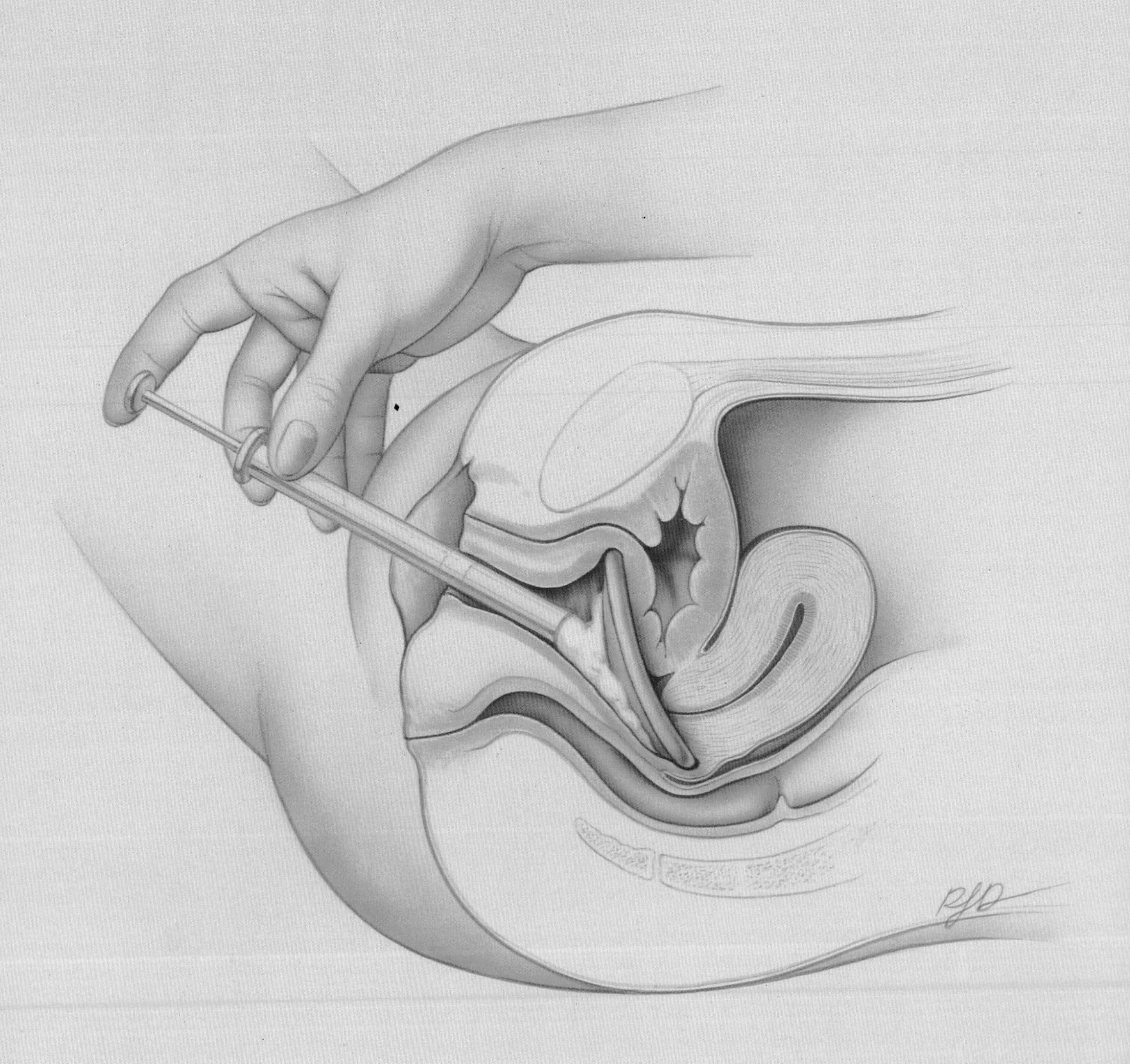

Hormonal Methods

Oral contraceptives, or birth-control pills, are perhaps the most popular form of birth control in the United States and the most effective method other than sterilization or abstinence. Today's birth-control pills are combinations of low-dose synthetic estrogen and progesterone. Very similar to the estrogen and progesterone that the woman produces in her ovaries and placenta, the synthetic hormones in the pill mimic a pregnancy in the woman who takes them. By elevating the levels of estrogen and progesterone in the woman's bloodstream, these pills artificially keep the levels of follicle-stimulating hormone (FSH) and luteinizing hormone (LH) very low. In the absence of LF and FSH, the ovarian follicle will not develop and an egg will not mature or be expelled from the ovary. If there is no ovulation, there can be no fertilization and no pregnancy.

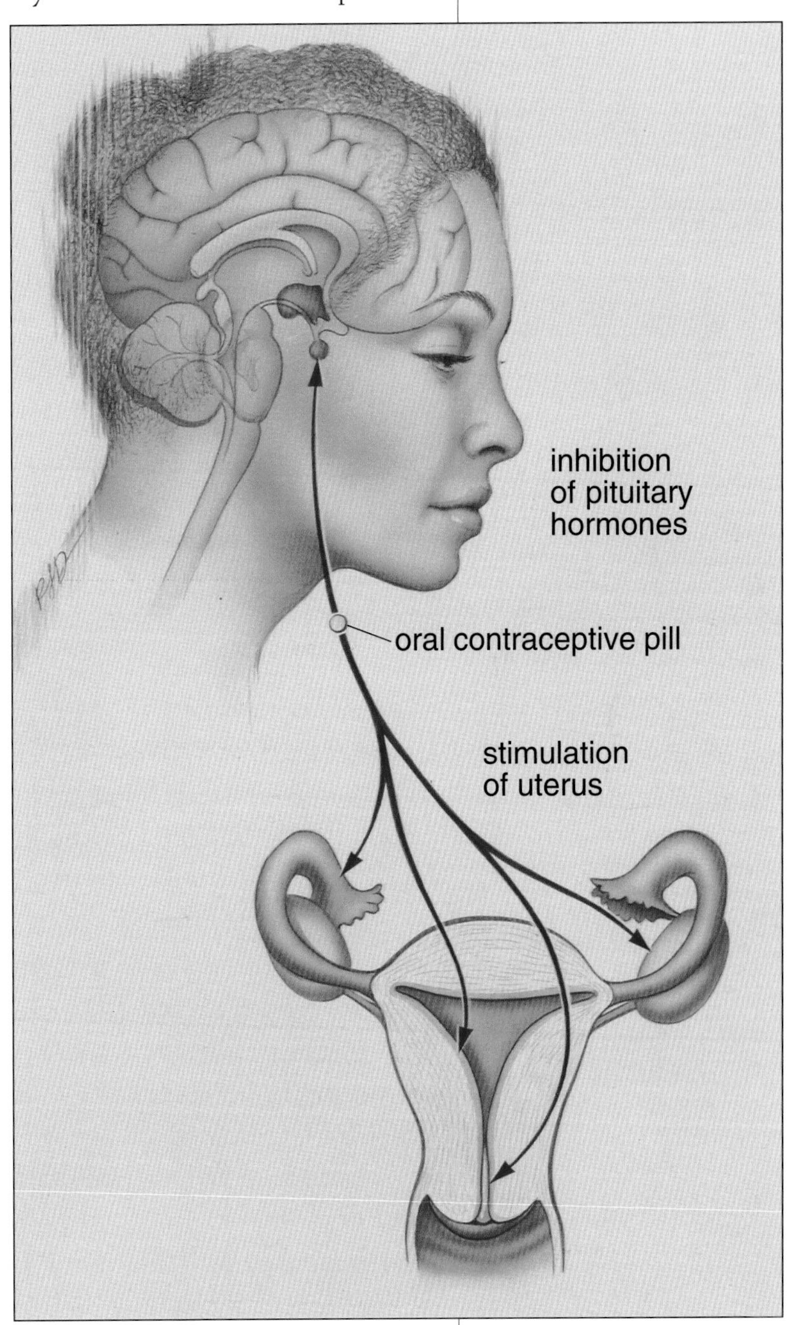

59. *Mode of Action of Oral Contraceptive*

In addition to suppressing ovulation, the birth control pill prevents pregnancy in other ways. If an egg does mature despite the oral contraceptive, it may have difficulty migrating down the Fallopian tube to the uterus. The hormonal pill seems to alter the normal contractions of the tube. There is little chance of sperm being available to fertilize the egg, because the birth control pill makes the cervical mucus particularly hostile to sperm cells trying to enter the uterus. And finally, if the egg is fertilized in the tube and reaches the uterus, the endometrium will not be prepared to

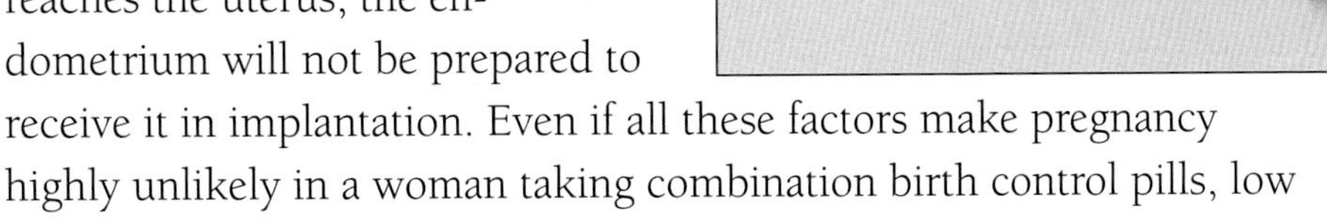
receive it in implantation. Even if all these factors make pregnancy highly unlikely in a woman taking combination birth control pills, low

failure rates are noted, probably because the pills are not taken as directed. Although the pills are meant to be taken every day for three weeks per month, many of the pill manufacturers package three weeks' worth of active pills and one week of sugar pills so that the woman need not interrupt pill-taking through a four-week cycle.

Some birth control pills that combine estrogen and progesterone have varying doses of progesterone throughout the month. Called phasic contraceptives, these combination pills also seem to control fertility with minimal side effects. A pure progesterone pill exists for women who are unable to take estrogen. Although progesterone alone does not prevent ovulation, it does alter the cervical mucus and the endometrium to limit fertilization and implantation and is moderately effective in preventing pregnancy.

In special cases, a birth control pill is taken after intercourse to try to prevent pregnancy. Mainly used in cases of rape occurring a few days before ovulation or as a back-up after a condom breaks, a combination of estrogen and progesterone at higher doses than exist in ordinary birth control pills is given. These post-coital or "morning-after" pills are able to prevent pregnancy in most cases.

60. Pills are Packaged in Many Different Dispensers. Reminders are Built into the Design to Keep the Patient on Schedule

Side effects of birth control pills may limit their use. Some women on the birth control pill experience some swelling, weight gain, mood changes, sleepiness, breast tenderness, nervousness, or acne. Smokers over the age of 35 are at increased risk for complications and should choose another method. Women with diabetes, history of stroke or heart disease, high blood pressure, breast cancer, endometrial cancer, or thrombophlebitis (blood clot formation) should not take birth control pills. Women who are nursing infants should not take the pill, as the hormones will enter the breast milk and may affect the infant.

The birth control pill confers a number of health benefits in addition to the ability to plan pregnancies. The pills appear to protect women who take them from endometrial and ovarian cancers and benign breast disease. Because periods are generally shorter and lighter while on the birth control pill, iron-deficiency anemia is not as common among women who take them.

Two additional methods exist for preventing pregnancy through hormonal means. In countries other than the United States, women can be treated with intermittent injections of progesterone. Some forms require injection monthly; others need to be administered only every three months. The progesterone prevents pregnancy by making the endometrium unable to sustain an implanted fertilized egg and by effects on the cervical mucus. However, the progesterones cause menstrual irregularities, and women sometimes need a year off the injections before their fertility returns.

A woman can also have progesterone implanted beneath her skin. Progesterone is absorbed into match-stick-sized pieces of plastic and slipped under the skin on the upper arm. These sticks remain in place for up to five years, slowly releasing progesterone and preventing the uterus and cervix from allowing a pregnancy. Sometimes, the implants can be difficult to remove.

Intrauterine Devices

Among the oldest forms of birth control, the intrauterine device (IUD) is an object inserted through the cervix and placed within the uterus to prevent pregnancy. IUDs can be made of metal, plastic, or other substances and have been manufactured in many different shapes. Scientists still do not fully understood how the IUD works.

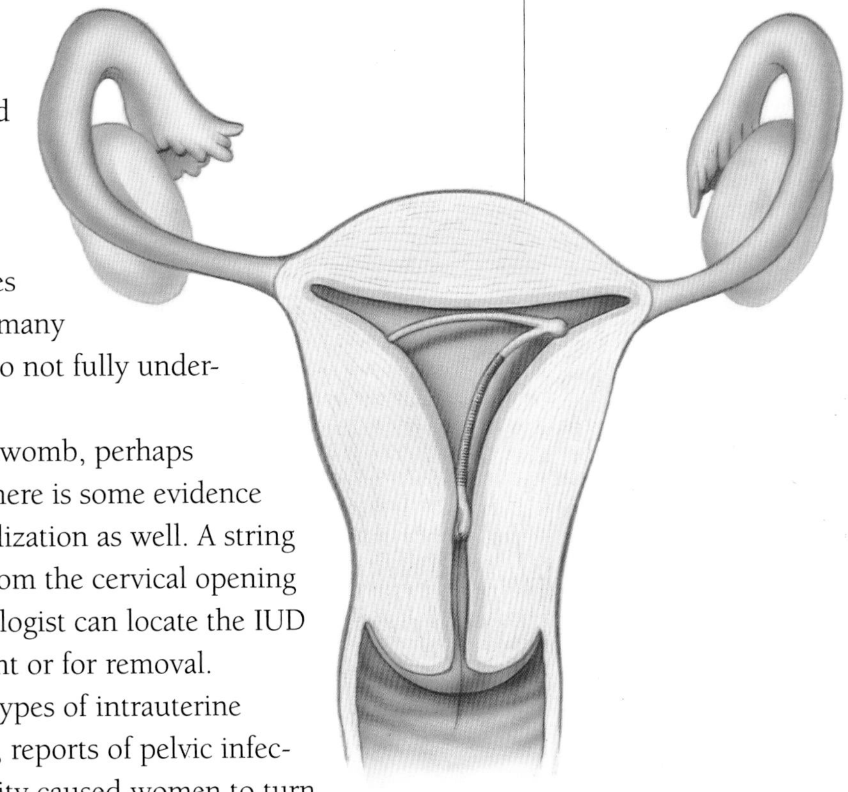

The IUD remains within the womb, perhaps interfering with implantation. There is some evidence that the IUD interferes with fertilization as well. A string attached to the IUD protrudes from the cervical opening so that a woman and her gynecologist can locate the IUD for assurance of proper placement or for removal.

Until the mid-1980s, many types of intrauterine devices were available. However, reports of pelvic infections, tubal infections, and sterility caused women to turn toward other methods. Multiple lawsuits in the United States have forced the manufacturers to remove most of the devices from sale. IUDs containing progesterone or copper are still available. Both these substances seem to decrease the risks of the IUD.

The side effects of the IUD include increased menstrual cramping and bleeding, the risk of uterine perforation while placing the IUD, increased rates of pelvic infection, loss of the IUD during a period, and increased risk of ectopic pregnancy. The advantages are the ease of birth control once the device is placed, the relatively high effectiveness of the method, and the usually prompt return of fertility once the device is removed.

61. Intrauterine Device in Place in Uterus

Surgical Methods of Sterilization

The methods of birth control discussed earlier–barrier methods, hormonal methods, and the intrauterine device–are reversible. Although the hormonal methods may have effects on the reproductive organs that last for months and the IUD can cause infections in the tubes which may limit fertility, on the whole these methods do not prevent pregnancy once the person stops using them. If a man or a woman desires to put an end to fertility forever, he or she seeks surgical sterilization. Special consent processes have been developed for the patient requesting sterilization to assure that the person has considered all aspects of the procedure and has freely chosen it. Women are asked to sign a consent at least a month prior to the actual operation, giving them some time to change their minds.

"Sterilization in both men and women entails the surgical cutting of an anatomical part of their body–the vas deferens in the man and the Fallopian tubes in the woman."

Sterilization in both men and women entails the surgical cutting of an anatomical part of their body–the vas deferens in the man and the Fallopian tubes in the woman. Sterility is virtually assured, although there are reports of the vas deferens or tube reattaching itself. Also, doctors are sometimes able to reverse the sterilization surgically in cases where a man or a woman changes his or her mind some time after the operation has been done and desires a pregnancy. Success of the repair, however, is not high and sterilization for either man or woman should not be performed on the patient uncertain of future plans for pregnancy. Worldwide, sterilization is the most widespread form of birth control practised.

VASECTOMY

The sterilization procedure in the man is a simple office procedure called a vasectomy. A urologist, a doctor who specializes in the care of the male genital and urinary systems, will numb a small area on both scrotal sacs. A small incision is then made in the skin on both sides and the vas deferens located. A short length of the tube, around a half-inch, is cut away entirely so that the ends of the tube will not touch, and the cut ends are tied. Cutting the vas deferens does not prevent sperm from being produced and does not interfere with the male hormones or their bodily effects. Nor does it interfere with sexual performance or pleasure. Instead, the sterilization procedure merely prevents the sperm from getting into the semen. When the man has an ejaculation after a vasectomy, his semen will contain everything except

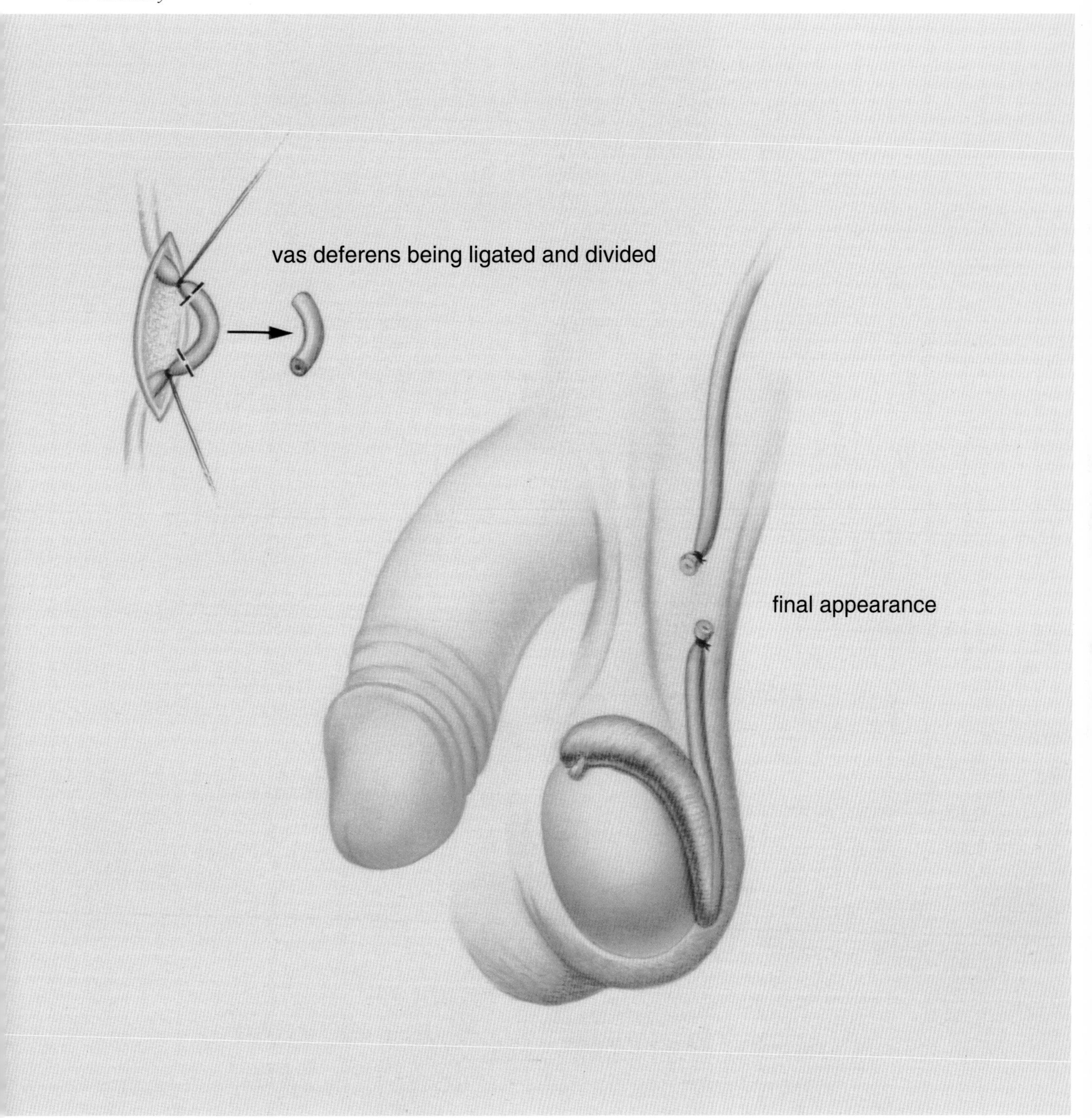
vas deferens being ligated and divided
final appearance

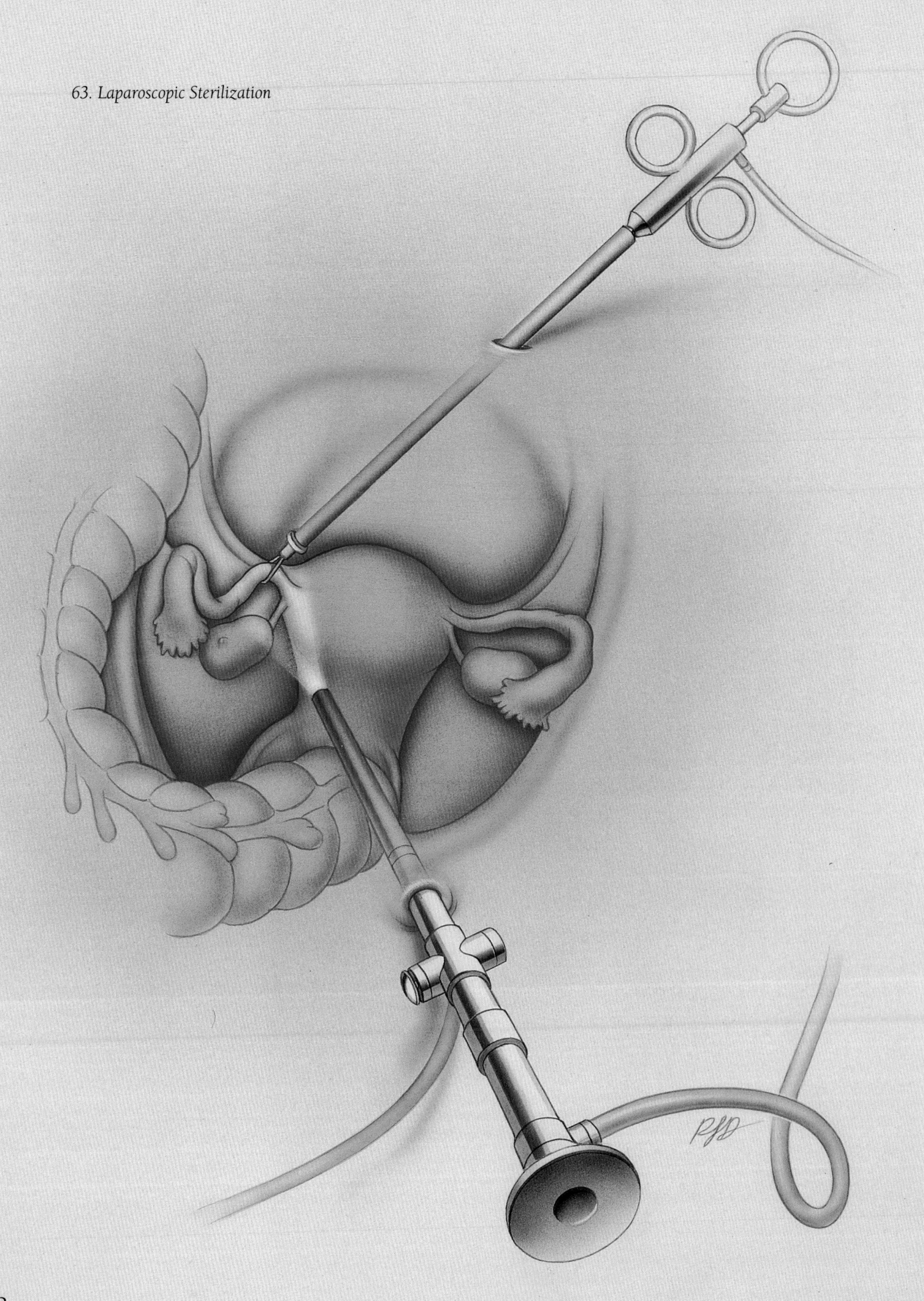

63. Laparoscopic Sterilization

the sperm. However, because sperm may be stored throughout the tube and seminal vesicles and near the glands, the man will not be fully sterile until several weeks after the procedure. By examining the semen some time after a vasectomy, the doctor can confirm when the sperm are completely removed from the semen.

Tubal Ligation

Sterilization for the woman is somewhat more complicated, although it, too, can be done without spending a night in the hospital. Because the reproductive organs requiring surgery are internal and not external like a man's, sterilizing the woman requires an abdominal operation or laparoscopic surgery, in which instruments are inserted into tiny incisions in the abdominal wall and manipulated with the help of special cameras and lenses.

The gynecologist performing a sterilization on a woman cuts, clips, or electrocoagulates both Fallopian tubes.

This procedure does not interfere with ovulation in the ovary but it does prevent the egg from traveling down the Fallopian tube, becoming fertilized, and implanting in the uterus.

Many surgical procedures exist for interrupting the Fallopian tube. A segment of each tube can be removed, a loop can be tied in each tube, or a silastic ring can be placed on the tubes.

The procedure must be done on both sides at once to be effective. There are few side effects known to the procedure, although some women report an increase in menstrual cramping or irregular periods after tubal ligation.

Both men and women may feel some regret after a sterilization procedure. A grief reaction is normal, for the man or woman has given up future children. However well considered and well justified, sterilization ordinarily has emotional consequences that the doctor and the patient should expect. These procedures do not affect libido or sexual performance, and some couples report an increase in pleasure and spontaneity in sexual activities once the danger of an unwanted pregnancy is removed.

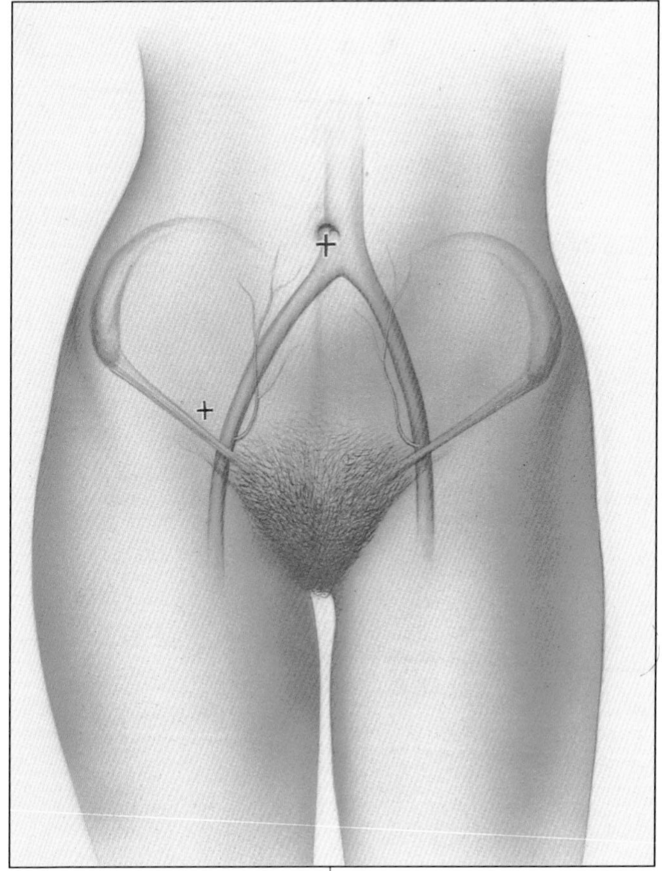

64. Sites of Small Incisions for Laparoscopic Sterilization

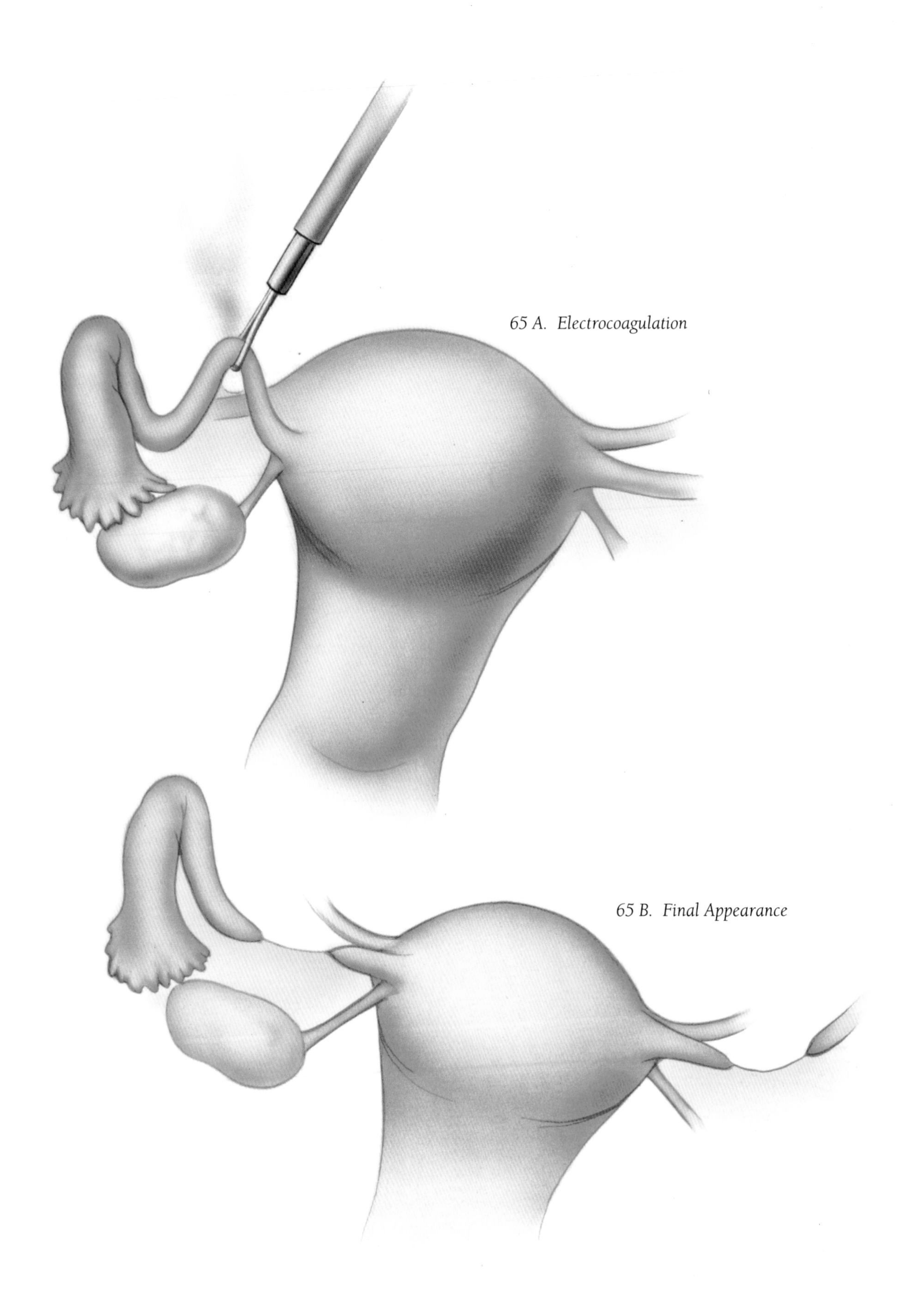
65 A. *Electrocoagulation*

65 B. *Final Appearance*

66. Tubal Ligation with Silastic Rings

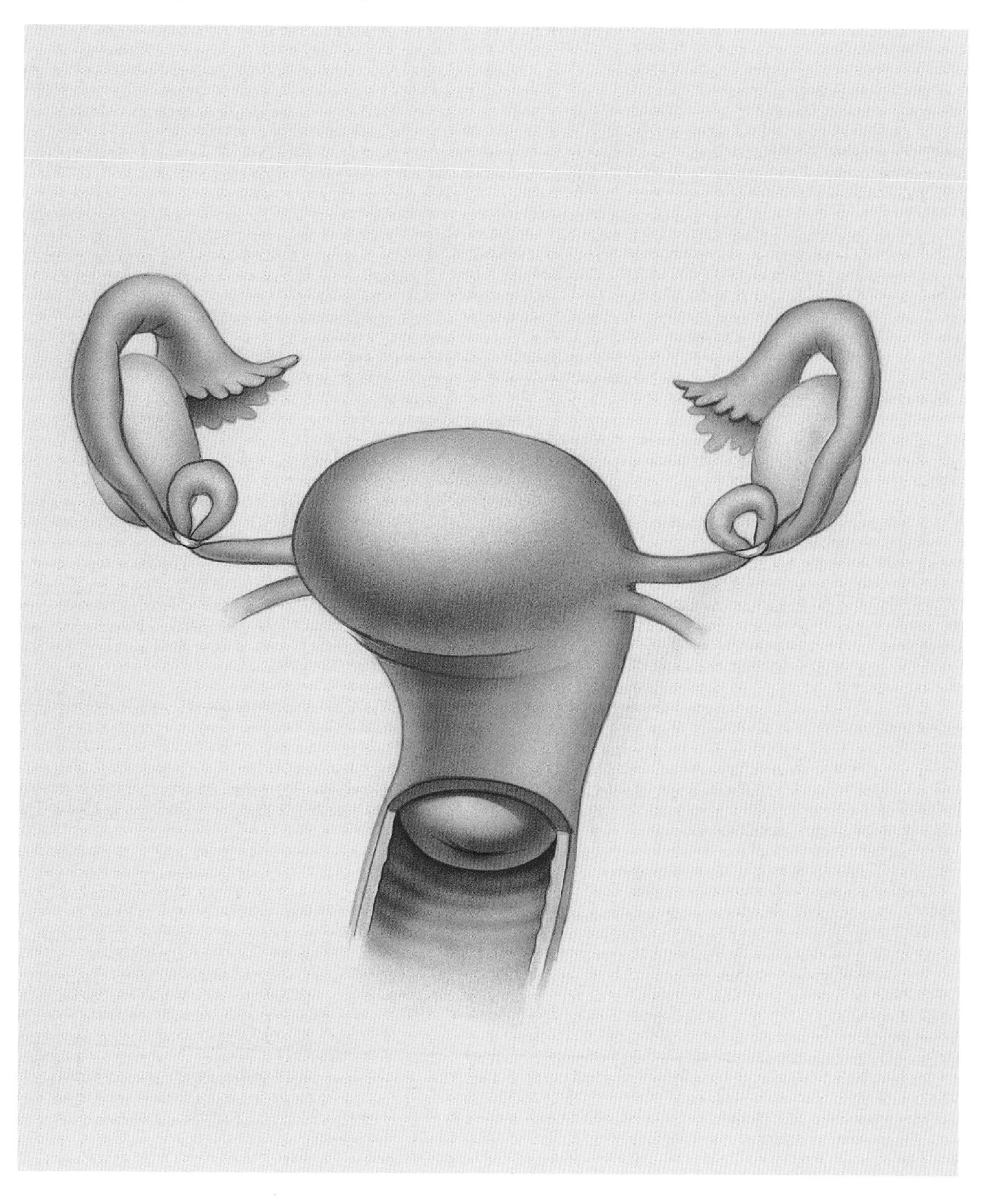

Man and Woman: Treatment of Infertility

"Approximately 15% of couples in developed countries may experience infertility, with the man and the woman contributing about equally to the cause of the problem."

Some couples find that they are unable to conceive a child. A couple is considered to be infertile if they have not conceived a child after a year of having intercourse regularly without birth control. Approximately 15% of couples in developed countries may experience infertility, with the man and the woman contributing equally to the causes of the problem. Such common practices as smoking cigarettes, using contraceptives, delaying pregnancy until older ages, and contraction of sexually transmitted diseases all can play a part in infertility. Often, more than one specific problem can be found in the infertile couple.

Any part of the complex process of reproduction in the man or in the woman–from production of the egg and the sperm, travel of the sperm to the Fallopian tube, fertilization, implantation, or maintenance of pregnancy–can be a factor in infertility. Gynecologists and urologists have made great progress in diagnosing the particular problems faced by an infertile couple. Treatments are available for many specific diagnoses, and couples sometimes get pregnant without treatment once an evaluation for infertility has been initiated. The couple seeking help in fertility will undergo a comprehensive evaluation, seeking treatable causes in both the male and the female partner.

Male Factors

The man's semen will be examined for adequacy and health of sperm cells. Infections, hormonal problems, anatomical abnormalities in the testicles or vas deferens, and antibody formation can all influence the ability of the sperm to fertilize an egg. Underlying medical problems such as diabetes or thyroid disease must be treated. Such simple changes in behavior as stopping smoking, stopping alcoholic drinking, avoiding exposure to high temperatures, and wearing only loose-fitting underclothes can sometimes solve the problem.

In some cases, surgery is required to repair abnormalities in the vas deferens or spermatic cord. Other treatments are available to increase sperm production and vigor. The sperm is sometimes unable to gain access to the uterus and the Fallopian tube for fertilization. In these cases, the doctors may offer the couple artificial insemination, a procedure of removing the man's semen from an ejaculated sample and inserting it directly into the woman's vagina or uterus.

FEMALE FACTORS

The woman will be fully examined with a pelvic examination and other specialized procedures as needed. Hormonal conditions, infections, antibody formation, anatomical problems of the cervix, uterus, or Fallopian tubes, exposure to diethylstilbestrol (DES), and ovulatory problems can all contribute to infertility.

Surgery can correct some of these problems. For example, removing a uterine fibroid tumor or repairing a damaged Fallopian tube can increase the woman's chance of becoming pregnant. Women with endometriosis, a condition in which endometrial tissue is found outside the uterus in the abdominal cavity, may require surgery or medical treatment. Such medical diseases as liver disease, thyroid problems, diabetes, kidney disease, and obesity are treated appropriately. Hormonal treatment is sometimes necessary for the woman to produce healthy cervical mucus. Infections in the pelvis can be treated with antibiotics. Some cases of infertility due to abnormal cervical mucus or antibody formation can be treated with artificial insemination using the sperm of the woman's partner.

Ovarian problems may demand more complex treatment by the gynecologist. In some women the ovaries are not able to develop a follicle in the monthly cycle. Although eggs are present in the ovary, the normal mechanisms that ordinarily lead to the monthly release of an egg are impaired. Many medical problems can cause such impairment.

The evaluation examines the ovulatory cycles by checking the basal body temperature and measuring the reproductive hormones at particular times in the cycle. Endometrial biopsies are sometimes used to pinpoint the problem to a particular stage of the ovulatory cycle. Ultrasound or laparoscopic examinations may be used to visualize the ovaries during the cycle.

Women who do not ovulate can be treated with hormones to encourage the development of eggs in the ovaries. Such medicines as estrogen, human chorionic gonadotropin, clomiphene or human menopausal gonadotropin are used separately or in sequence to stimulate eggs to mature. The gynecologist tailors the medical treatment to each individual patient's particular problem, checking with ultrasound examinations or blood tests to determine the effectiveness of the treatment. These hormonal treatments will often stimulate multiple egg production, increasing the possibilities of having twins, triplets, or even more babies at once.

"Some cases of infertility due to abnormal cervical mucus or antibody formation can be treated with artificial insemination using the sperm of the woman's partner."

In Vitro Fertilization

There are cases in which hormonal treatments alone will not lead to pregnancy, either because the egg cannot travel to the Fallopian tube or cannot join with the sperm. In vitro fertilization (IVF) has been developed for such cases. In this expensive and complex procedure, the woman's ovaries are stimulated with hormonal treatment to produce eggs. At the proper time in the ovulatory cycle, the gynecologist uses a needle guided by ultrasound, or, in rare instances, a laparoscopic procedure, to remove eggs from the ovary. The eggs are fertilized with sperm in the laboratory, using her partner's sperm, if healthy, or donor sperm. After two to three days of growth, one or more fertilized eggs are placed back into the woman's uterus. Fertilized eggs are sometimes frozen for use during a future cycle.

"At the proper time in the ovulatory cycle, the gynecologist uses a needle guided by ultrasound, or, in rare instances, a laparoscopic procedure, to remove eggs from the ovary."

If a woman cannot produce her own eggs even with hormonal treatment, she can undergo donor egg implantation. In this procedure, another woman allows the eggs to be removed from her ovary. These eggs are fertilized in the laboratory using the potential father's sperm and implanted into the uterus of the woman desiring pregnancy. Alternatively, the donor woman is artificially inseminated, using sperm of the partner of the woman desiring pregnancy. Three to four days later, the uterus of the donor woman is rinsed, hoping to obtain a fertilized egg from the lining of her uterus. This fertilized egg is then implanted into the uterus of the woman desiring pregnancy. Although the baby born of such a pregnancy will not be the genetic child of the pregnant woman, it will develop in her uterus for a full term pregnancy. Many questions arise about the rights and responsibilities of the persons involved in such pregnancies. Nonetheless, these new techniques are bringing hope to infertile couples who earlier would have had no chance for a pregnancy.

Throughout the evaluation and treatment for infertility, couples routinely require psychological support. The procedures can be exhausting, expensive, and stressful on all aspects of the couple's life. Support groups exist to help couples through the highs and lows of pregnancy attempts. Although some couples choose adoption or childlessness, the majority of couples seeking infertility treatments are able to conceive.

On the Woman's Side: Menopause

The menstrual cycles gradually stop as a woman reaches her late forties or early fifties. Called menopause, the stopping of the periods is due to the drop in estrogen production and egg formation in the ovaries. This normal period in a woman's life brings both benefits and problems. Although many uncertainties still exist, doctors and scientists are working hard to learn about the effects of menopause on the woman's body and the best way to treat women following menopause.

EFFECTS OF MENOPAUSE

The most significant benefit of menopause is the freedom from the worry of unwanted pregnancy. Because they are no longer fertile, women after menopause can stop using contraceptives. Some women experience increased spontaneity of sexual activity, freed from the necessity to keep track of fertile periods of the cycle or to interrupt sexual play for diaphragm insertion. Untreated, menopause also ends the monthly bleeding cycle, a minor benefit to women who have suffered with their periods.

Estrogen and progesterone levels drop after menopause. Because the reproductive hormones influence the woman's body in many ways, a drop in their levels has predictable effects. The vaginal lining becomes thinner and smoother, and cervical mucus and vaginal lubrication decrease. The breasts may decrease slightly in size. Skin all over the body can lose some elasticity. Hot flushes, in which women become warm and sweaty even in cool environments, occur commonly, sometimes associated with heart palpitations or feelings of dizziness or weakness.

The dropping levels of hormones have effects that the woman cannot see or feel. Although the research is still not conclusive, heart disease may become more common in women after menopause because the hormones seem to protect the arteries and appear to benefit a woman's cholesterol levels. Bone strength can decline in the absence of estrogen, giving women risks for fractures of the hip or vertebral bones, usually around ten years after menopause.

"Hot flushes, in which women become warm and sweaty even in cool environments, occur commonly, sometimes associated with heart palpitations or feelings of dizziness or weakness."

67. Female Reproductive Organs Following the Menopause (actual size)

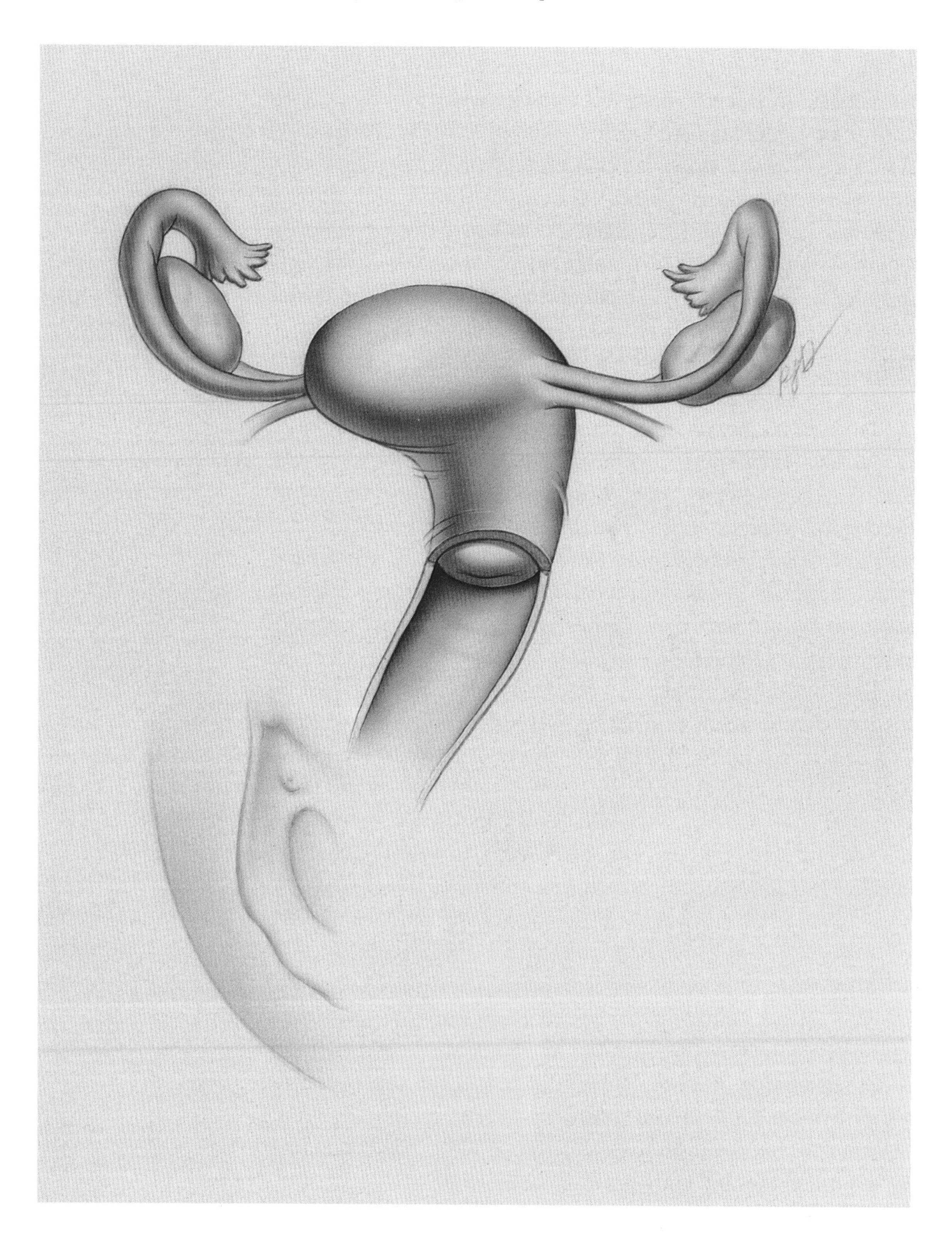

Hormonal Replacement Therapy

Estrogen replacement is becoming more common in view of the potential medical benefits derived. Carefully prescribed by a doctor, hormone replacement may protect a woman from heart disease or bone disease, although some risk is involved. Because taking estrogen alone can increase a woman's risk of endometrial cancer, doctors usually prescribe a combination of estrogen and progesterone to women who have not had the uterus removed. Endometrial biopsies will be done regularly to check on the side effects of the hormone treatments. Since women on replacement hormones may be at added risk for breast cancer, they should be followed closely with breast examinations and mammograms. Women who take estrogen and progesterone combinations may resume their monthly periods, although their fertility does not return. Replacement hormones must be continued for the rest of the woman's life.

There are instances in which women should not take replacement hormones, including certain types of liver disease, breast disease, uterine disease, and blood clotting problems. Side effects of the hormone treatments may include increase in blood pressure, thrombophlebitis, diabetes, and migraine headache. The decision to embark on long-term hormone replacement therapy is an individual choice, made by each woman in consultation with her doctor. As more becomes known about both the benefits and the risks of hormone replacement treatment, women and their doctors can make increasingly informed choices.

"Carefully prescribed by a doctor, hormone replacement may protect a woman from heart disease or bone disease, although some risk is involved."

Man and Woman: Sexually Active Forever

"Many couples find that in menopause, when they need not worry about birth control or unwanted pregnancy, they become even more able to enjoy each other sexually."

Because a couple can no longer conceive a child does not mean their sexual lives are over. Many couples find that in menopause, when they need not worry about birth control or unwanted pregnancy, they become even more able to enjoy each other sexually. Although some of the physiological changes of menopause may hinder sexual pleasure, these are easily remedied. Men can conceive children their entire lives, for the sperm continue to be produced in the testicles–although in lower and lower numbers–until the man's death. The post-menopausal woman can conceive a child only with the help of high technology and hormone replacement.

Studies of older men and women confirm the belief that sexual pleasures can continue as long as reasonably good health is present. Doctors are becoming sensitive to older couples' sexual desires, and should make sure to ask their older patients about their enjoyment of sex. Sexual closeness adds pleasure and depth to a shared life, bringing couples together throughout their lives in physical and emotional intimacy.

Glossary

AFTERBIRTH. *The placenta and fetal membranes expelled after delivery of the baby.*
AMNION. *A thin, transparent membranous sac which forms the inner wall of the fetal membranes and which holds the fetus suspended in fluid.*
"BAG OF WATERS." *The fetal membranes. See amnion.*
BASAL BODY TEMPERATURE GRAPH (BBT). *A graph which records the daily body temperature of the female. A rise in temperature indicates that ovulation has occurred.*
BIRTH CONTROL. *Any method used to control pregnancy.*
BLASTOCYST. *A stage in the development of an embryo. In this stage, the embryo consists of a layer of cells surrounding a fluid-filled cavity.*
BULBOURETHRAL GLANDS. *Two small glands located on each side of the prostate gland. They secrete a fluid forming part of the seminal fluid. Also called Cowper's glands.*
CALENDAR RHYTHM METHOD. *A contraceptive technique which allows intercourse during that period of the menstrual cycle when ovulation is not likely to occur. This technique uses calendar days for calculation.*
CERVICAL CAP. *A device placed over the cervix to prevent conception.*
CERVICAL MUCUS. *An adhering, slippery secretion of the cervix.*
CERVIX. *The narrow, outer end of the uterus resembling a neck.*
CESAREAN SECTION. *The delivery of a baby by way of a surgical incision of the walls of the abdomen and uterus.*
"CHANGE OF LIFE." *See menopause.*
CHORION. *The outer layer of the fetal membranes which serves as a protective and nutritive covering for the fertilized egg, the developing embryo, and the fetus.*
CHORIONIC GONADOTROPIN. *A hormone produced by the placenta which stimulates the corpus luteum of the ovary to produce progesterone.*
CHORIONIC SAC OR VESICLE. *See chorion.*
CHROMOSOMES. *Small rod-shaped bodies present in the cell nucleus which contain hereditary factors.*
CIRCUMCISION. *The removal of the foreskin of the glans penis.*
CLITORIS. *A small organ located at the anterior of the external female genital organs.*
COITUS. *Sexual intercourse between persons of the opposite sex.*
COITUS INTERRUPTUS. *Withdrawal of the penis from the vagina before the ejaculation of semen.*
COMBINATION PILLS. *Birth control pills that contain two synthetic hormones (estrogen and progesterone) in the same tablet. When these pills are used, the endometrium and cervical mucus approximate the condition that they would have during the postovulatory phase of the menstrual cycle.*
CONCEPTION. *The union of the sperm and the egg, which results in pregnancy.*
CONDOM. *A covering worn over the penis during intercourse to prevent pregnancy.*
CONTRACEPTION. *The voluntary prevention of conception or pregnancy.*
CORPUS LUTEUM. *A yellow mass in the ovary formed by an ovarian follicle that has matured and discharged its egg.*
COWPER'S GLAND. *See bulbourethral glands.*
DELIVERY. *Passage of the baby through the birth canal.*
DIAPHRAGM. *A rubber or plastic cup which fits over the cervix and is used for contraceptive purposes.*
DOUCHE. *A hygienic procedure consisting of passing a stream of solution into the vagina.*
DYSMENORRHEA. *Painful or uncomfortable menstruation.*
ECTOPIC PREGNANCY. *The abnormal implantation of the fertilized egg outside the uterine cavity.*
EGG. *A female cell capable of developing into a new member of the species.*

Ejaculation. *The expulsion of semen from the male urethra.*

Ejaculatory Ducts. *The terminal portion of the duct through which sperm are conveyed to the urethra.*

Embryo. *The stage of early development when the organs of the body are being formed.*

Emission. *A discharge of semen into the urethra.*

Endometrium. *The tissue layer lining the inner surface of the uterus.*

Epididymis. *An elongated structure at the back of the testes, in which the sperm are matured and stored.*

Episiotomy. *Surgical incision of the vulva during childbirth.*

Erectile Tissue. *Vascular tissue which, when filled with blood, becomes erect or rigid, such as the clitoris or penis.*

Erection. *The state of swelling, hardness, and stiffness observed in the penis, and to a lesser extent in the clitoris, due to sexual excitement.*

Estrogen. *A female sex hormone produced by the ovarian follicle which stimulates the internal female reproductive organs and the development of secondary sex characteristics in the female.*

Fallopian Tube. *The tube or duct which extends laterally from the uterus, terminating near the ovary. It conducts the egg from the ovary to the uterus and the sperm from the uterus toward the ovary.*

Fertile Period. *That period during which the female is most apt to become pregnant.*

Fertilization. *The union of sperm and egg.*

Fetus. *An unborn child between the fourteenth week of pregnancy and birth.*

Foreskin. *Loose skin at and covering the end of the penis.*

Fraternal Twins. *Twins which are the product of two separate fertilized eggs and are not identical.*

Genital. *Relating to the organs of reproduction in both the male and female.*

Glans Penis. *Bulbous end or head of the penis in which the urethral orifice is located.*

Gonads. *The female sex glands or ovaries and the male sex glands or testes.*

Gonadotropic Hormones. *See gonadotropin.*

Gonadotropin. *A hormone which stimulates the sex glands.*

Hormone. *A chemical substance produced by a gland and carried by the bloodstream to another area of the body where it exerts its effect.*

Hymen. *A thin ring of tissue partly closing the vaginal opening.*

Hypothalamus. *The area of the brain adjacent to the pituitary gland.*

Identical Twins. *Twins which are the product of one single fertilized egg and are of the same genetic makeup and sex.*

Implantation. *Attaching and embedding of the blastocyst into the uterine wall.*

Introitus. *The opening of the vagina.*

Intrauterine Device (IUD/IUCD). *A plastic or metal device inserted in the uterus as a means of contraception.*

Labia Majora. *The two rounded folds on either side of the vulva.*

Labia Minora. *The two thin folds of skin lying on either side of the vulva between the labia majora and the opening of the vagina.*

Labor. *The physiological process by which the fetus is expelled by the uterus at time of birth.*

Lactation. *The secretion of milk from the female's breasts.*

Lactogen. *A hormone which stimulates the secretion of milk.*

Luteinizing Hormone. *A gonadotropic hormone which is secreted by the pituitary gland and causes the ovarian follicle to rupture and release an egg.*

Maturation. *The process of becoming mature.*

Menopause. *That period which marks the permanent stoppage of ovarian and menstrual activity.*

Menstrual Cycle. *The reproductive cycle of the human female characterized by a recurrent series of changes in the uterus and sex organs.*

Menstrual Extraction. *Aspiration of the endometrial lining with a hand-held vacuum syringe, usually performed shortly after a missed menstrual period. This is the same as menstrual regulation or endometrial extraction.*

Menstruation. *The periodic discharge of a bloody fluid from the uterus into the vagina at regular intervals during the menstrual cycle.*

Mid-Trimester. *The middle three months of pregnancy.*

Mini-Pills. *An oral chemical agent still in the experimental phase which affects the cervical mucus and blocks sperm penetration.*

Mittelschmerz. *Pain between menstrual periods, associated with ovulation .*

Morula. *An early stage in development during which the fertilized egg consists of a solid mass of cells, resembling a mulberry.*

Nutrient. *Food for the body.*

Nocturnal Emission. *Spontaneous ejaculation during sleep.*

Oral Contraceptive. *A method of preventing conception based on oral medication or pills.*

Orgasm. *A state of excitement which occurs during sexual intercourse.*

Ovarian Follicles. *A spherical structure in the ovary consisting of an egg and its surrounding cells.*

Ovaries. *Two glands in the female producing the eggs and hormones.*

Oviducts. *Two tubes extending from the uterus which convey the egg from the ovary to the uterus. See Fallopian tube.*

Ovulation. *The ripening of the mature ovarian follicle and the release of the egg.*

Oxytocin. *A pituitary hormone which stimulates contraction of the uterine musculature to expel the fetus.*

Pelvis. *The bones of lower portion of the trunk of the body.*

Penis. *The male organ of reproduction.*

Perineum. *The area at the base of the body between the thighs.*

Pituitary Gland. *A small structure at the base of the brain which secretes hormones.*

Pituitary Hormone. *A hormone secreted by the pituitary gland.*

Placenta. *The oval spongy structure in the uterus through which the fetus derives its nourishment. Major component of the afterbirth.*

Polar Body. *One of two minute cells given off successively by the egg during its development.*

Postcoital Pills. *A means of contraception with pills taken after intercourse.*

Postovulation *That period after ovulation.*

Postpartum Period. *That period after the birth of the baby until the mother's body returns to its prepregnant condition.*

Pregnancy. *The condition of being with child.*

Premature Infant. *A child born before full development.*

Preovulation. *The period before ovulation.*

Prepuce. *The fold of skin that covers the end of the penis or the glans penis.*

Progesterone. *A female sex hormone produced by the corpus luteum of the ovary.*

Prostate Gland. *A gland located around the male urethra, which secretes a thin fluid that forms part of the semen.*

Puberty. *That time of life when the male or female becomes capable of reproduction.*

Reproduction. *The process which gives rise to offspring.*

Reproductive System. *The organs in the male and female that are utilized in the role of creating new life.*

Rhythm Method. *A contraceptive method which allows sexual intercourse only during the time of the menstrual cycle that the female is least susceptible to fertilization.*

"Safe" Period. *The time during the menstrual cycle when the female is least fertile.*

Scrotum. *The skin pouches beneath the penis containing the testicles.*

Semen. *A thick milky secretion composed of sperm and seminal fluid.*

Seminal Pool. *The deposit of semen in the vagina.*

SEMINAL VESICLES. *Sac-like structures in the male which secrete a thick fluid that forms part of the semen.*

SEQUENTIAL PILLS. *An oral contraceptive medication packaged so that the woman receives estrogen for three-quarters of her cycle and estrogen and progesterone for the remainder. This type of pill produces activity in the endometrium that parallels the normal cycle.*

SEXUAL INTERCOURSE. *Union of the male and female in which the penis is introduced into the vagina.*

SPERM. *The male fertilizing cell.*

SPERMICIDAL PREPARATION. *A chemical substance that will kill or immobilize sperm.*

SPERMATOCYTE. *A cell which will give rise to spermatozoa.*

SPERMATOGENESIS. *The formation of mature functioning sperm in the testes.*

SPERMATOZOA. *See sperm.*

STERILIZATION. *A procedure whereby a male or female is rendered incapable of reproduction. See tubal ligation and vasectomy.*

SYNTHETIC HORMONE. *A chemical manufactured artificially to approximate that produced naturally.*

TEMPERATURE RHYTHM METHOD. *A contraceptive technique which allows intercourse during that period of the menstrual cycle when ovulation is not likely to occur. This technique uses basal body temperature for calculation. See basal body temperature graph.*

TERM FETUS. *An unborn child between thirty-eight and forty weeks of pregnancy.*

TESTES. *The male reproductive glands located in the scrotal sacs and which produce sperm and the hormone testosterone.*

TESTOSTERONE. *The principal male hormone which accelerates the development of secondary sexual characteristics. It is essential for normal sexual behavior and is responsible for the deepening of the male voice, muscle development, and growth of beard and pubic hair.*

TRIMESTER. *A period of three months. A full-term pregnancy of nine months is divided into three trimesters.*

TROPHOBLAST. *The outer layers of a developing fertilized egg that will become the placenta and fetal membranes.*

TUBAL LIGATION. *Female sterilization in which the Fallopian tubes are cut and the middle section usually removed.*

UMBILICAL CORD. *The cord connecting the fetus with the placenta.*

URETHRA. *The canal that discharges urine.*

URINARY BLADDER. *The receptacle that holds the urine before it is excreted.*

URINARY MEATUS. *The external opening of the urethra.*

UTERINE LINING. *The tissue covering the inside of the womb.*

UTERUS. *The muscular organ of the female which houses the fetus. Also known as the womb.*

VAGINA. *The canal extending from the vulva to the cervix.*

VAS DEFERENS. *The duct from the testes that carries the sperm.*

VAS LIGATION. *See vasectomy.*

VASECTOMY. *Male sterilization which involves surgical cutting of the vas deferens to cause permanent sterility.*

VERNIX CASEOSA. *A fatty secretion covering the fetus, most prevalent in the creases and folds of the skin.*

VULVA. *External parts of the female genital organs.*

WITHDRAWAL. *The removal of the penis from the vagina before ejaculation in order to prevent introduction of semen into the female.*

WOMB. *See uterus.*

ZONA PELLUCIDA. *A layer of material surrounding the egg through which the sperm must pass before fertilization can take place.*